When I was a little girl I had occasional bouts of the hiccups. Once they started it seemed no matter what I did I couldn't get rid of them. My mother said, "Here, let me give you a little MAGIC". She filled a glass with water and told me to bend over and drink the water upside down.
Guess what? My hiccups disappeared!

Moral of the story: sometimes a little 'magic' works!

Also by Anne Seifert:

Dr. Anne Good Health at Hand (Expanded Edition): Your lifelong way to eat, exercise and meditate Varnes Publishers, 2023, ISBN: 9780943584065

Dr. Anne Good Health at Hand (Quick Start): Your lifelong way to eat, exercise and meditate. Varnes Publishers, 2020, ISBN: 9780943584041

Contributor, To Be With God: Despite limitations of the brain, by Edward A.Siegel, M.D. CreateSpace, 2010

Magic-Hand Eating Plan: Good health, happiness and weight control. Varnes Publishers, 2004 ISBN:9780943584034

Contributor, Voices of Survival: In the nuclear age, by Dennis Paulson, Capra Press, 1986

The Intelligent Woman's Diet: The practical way to keep trim, relax, and stay well the rest of your life. Varnes Publishers, 1982 ISBN:0943584010

His, Mine, & Ours: A guide to keeping marriage from ruining a perfectly good relationship. Macmillan Publishing Company: 1979 ISBN:0026090309

Anne Seifert books available through online & other bookstores.

dr Anne plan

MANUAL & PRACTICE

The Handbook for
Good Health, Happiness & Weight Control™

Anne Seifert, M.P.H., Ph.D

Varnes Publishers

Seal Beach, California

dr.Anne is a registered trademark (USPTO).
Varnes Publishers
Seal Beach, CA 90740
varnespubs@email.com

Library of Congress Cataloging in Publication Data

Seifert, Anne M.
dr. Anne Plan MANUAL & PRACTICE: Good Health, Happiness & Weight Control

ISBN:978-0-943584-00-3

1. Health & Fitness 2. Diet & Nutrition 3. Weight Loss

Library of Congress Control Number: 2025936888

Printed in United States of America

Disclaimer:
The purpose of this book is to educate the reader about well-balanced nutrition and to provide a lifelong food-based portion-control program for good health and weight control. Individual results may vary. There is no guarantee as to how much weight will be lost following this program. The instruction given will for most people improve their general nutrition, health, and foster gradual safe weight loss.
It is offered with the understanding that each person is different, and it is the responsibility of the individual to check first with a health professional if there is any concern that the advice included herein might not apply for a specific situation or medical condition. Every effort has been made to make this a flexible and adaptable program. Readers are urged to tailor this information-- how to eat, exercise and meditate-- to meet their individual needs
Simply stated, know your own body and use your common sense when changing lifestyle habits.

dr Anne® Association

Mission Statement:
The Association's purpose is to provide public benefit educational programs, promote sustainable lifestyle change, reduce obesity, and enhance the enjoyment of life through flexible and research informed strategies. Based on decades of National Institutes of Health studies, these recommended health practices are associated with good health and increased longevity. We offer a flexible program adaptable to medical restrictions with a personalized approach to achieve wellness, empowerment, and spiritual growth. The Association is a volunteer-based, self-sustaining non-profit 501(c)(3) organization. Funds generated from the sale of program materials, donations, and courses are used to support the website, volunteer activities, and on-going Practice Circles. Learn more at www.dranne.org.

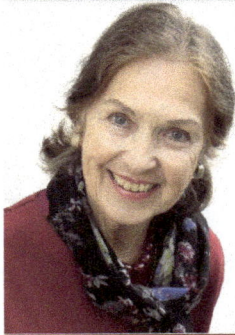

from the founder
Anne Seifert. M.P.H.. Ph.D.

We must consider that each one of us is unique. Like fingerprints no two are alike. For this reason what might be good for one person may not be good for another. Epidemiologists are the research arm of public health. Our solutions tend to be broad based to solve a population problem. As such, this plan intervenes at a practical level providing a health strategem while also accommodating personal preferences.

This practical Plan is inspired by Dr. Anne Seifert's NIH funded research to discover how healthy people stay healthy. After years of investigation what we suspected was true: sensible eating, moderate exercise, sleeping well, and maintaining body weight are all associated with well-being. This confirmed the landmark study conducted in the 1960's by Belloc and Breslow that lifestyle choices count. That study stood on the shoulders of research from the 1920's and 30's, and other studies followed. Started in 1976 the Nurse's Health Study continues to today-- with similar conclusions. Yes, a diet with fruits, vegetables, whole grains, unsaturated fats, nuts, legumes and low-fat dairy contribute to health, and reduce significantly the risk of many chronic diseases. Eating healthy remains key. And lifestyle impacts how well you will live.

What was surprising was how few people were able to change their behavior to achieve the goal of good health practices. Responsible programs for weight-loss and exercise were often too demanding. Dr. Anne reasoned that if she could find a way to make nutritious well-balanced eating easy and exercise enjoyable, perhaps more people would do it. Not only would people feel better, but they'd also lose weight and reduce the risk of diseases often attributed to old age, including heart disease, diabetes, and cancer.

She observed that one major culprit eroding good health is excess weight. The MagicHand eating approach was developed in 1980 to be permissive, allowing people to still include their favorite foods albeit in moderation for a lifetime of healthy eating. Other dally practices were also essential—exercise and meditation— completing this overall good health package.

Her first book on the program was published in 1982. The first public workshop introducing the hand as a portion measurer took place on February 6, 1984 for the City of Escondido.

To my beautiful sister

Louise

Thank you.

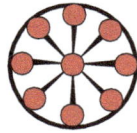

Focus Point	Table of Contents	Page

MANUAL

Apportion

Move

Silence

PRACTICE

Appendices

FOREWARD

In a world where health and weight management often feel like an uphill battle, my friend and colleague Dr. Anne Seifert offers a refreshing, doable, and practical approach to lasting wellness. Dr. Anne brings not only scientific expertise but also a compassionate, real-world perspective to the challenge of maintaining a healthy lifestyle.

Everything Dr. Anne does is rooted in research. As a co-investigator of a National Institutes of Health-funded study involving over 2,000 participants, she sought to understand the key factors that help people stay healthy. Her findings underscored a crucial truth: most chronic and debilitating diseases are either exacerbated or directly caused by excess weight. This realization inspired her to develop a weight-loss program that is not just effective but also flexible, fun and livable—a program designed for a lifetime of health. I am actively following her advice, and I can tell you, it works!

With a distinguished career as a researcher in the Department of Nutrition at Harvard University and as a member of the California Governor's Council on Wellness and Physical Fitness, Dr. Anne combines the rigor of science with a deep understanding of human behavior. Holding an M.A. in Psychology from Smith College and a doctorate in public health epidemiology from the University of California at Berkeley, she bridges the gap between research and practical application, making her insights both accessible and actionable.

The goal Dr. Anne's clever plan is clear: to promote balanced eating for effective weight control, to make the process interactive and enjoyable, and to encourage life-long changes in the realm of diet, exercise, and meditation.

What I love especially about her program is that is eschews rigid rules and mandates, and instead empowers us with the knowledge and tools we need to maintain a healthy weight in a way that fits into our normal, daily lives.

If you have struggled with weight management or simply want to take control of your health in a way that feels natural and sustainable, this book is for you.

Here's to a healthier, happier you, thanks to Dr. Anne!

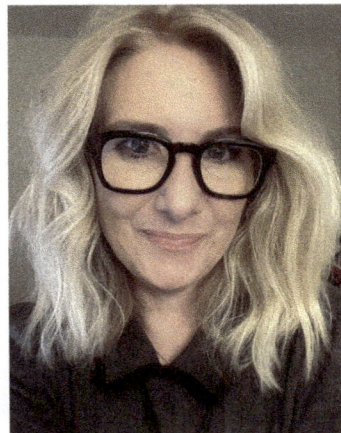

--Robin H. Phillips
Integrative Health Practitioner
Costa Mesa, CA

MANUAL

The word *Practice*:
To do or perform frequently— to create a habit.
It is also the act of continually doing something in order to get better at it.

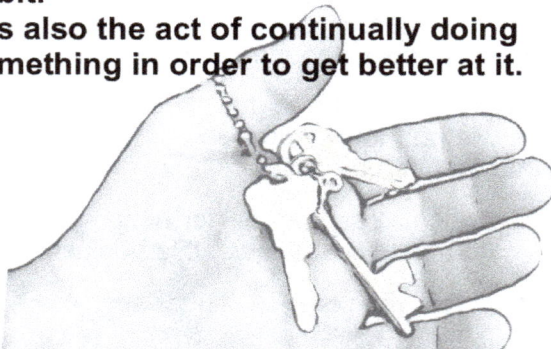

- **An example of practice is when you play the piano for 1/2 hour every day to become a better piano player.**

Introduction
Three Keys to Good Health

As an epidemiologist, I studied the risk factors predisposing one to disease. It is clear from my years of research that lifestyle counts. Good health practices mitigate many chronic diseases. The master key is lifestyle behavior. Clearly, being overweight exacerbates most chronic diseases. This book focuses on keeping your weight under control, staying active, and also finding quiet time. In short, this is a training course on how to live well.

How often have you heard that diets don't work? Well, for the most part, they do! The problem with most restrictive diet regimens is that they are too difficult to incorporate into one's life. Some people are able to live with "no-fat" diets, others can abstain from all sugar— they are rare, committed, disciplined people and I applaud them. Many still want a brownie.

Changing habits and finding your own way is the challenge. Imagine that you are about to learn how to play the violin. Someone hands you this instrument, already formed from wood with a bridge and strings and a bow. The objective is to be able to play pleasing music. But first you must learn how. Just as you must learn good health practices.

Your instrument is your body and it came with already set genes and predispositions. Learning the sheet music, and getting that violin to perform as it should requires PRACTICE.

Learning to make music requires coordination between the instrument and player. Practice, Practice, Practice. It does not stop. What musician, even when a virtuoso, stops practicing? And that's what you must do. Never stop practicing to keep good health habits in place. Here is the sheet music, the blueprint, for good health. Keep in mind that perhaps not every day will you be perfect, you may miss a note. It only means you must keep *practicing*.

This book is divided starting with an educational MANUAL and following with a self-help PRACTICE section that corresponds to the Points in the three keys to good health:

APPORTION	how to keep healthy weight control.
MOVE	how to find joyful exercising.
SILENCE	how to use meditation to visualize results.

Each key contains three Point chapters for lifelong well being— staying in tune. Going to the Practice section for each Point will personalize your journey to good health.

Why I wrote this book

Anyone who is overweight and wants to lose weight knows the exquisite misery of facing the mirror and asking, "How did this happen to me?" Skirts and slacks are too tight. What you wore last summer to the beach doesn't look as good this year. You contemplate whether it's time to go on a diet. Your friends are losing weight right and left on liquid diets and two-week wonder wafers, or drugs and you think that that's what to do. Just get the weight off. Then you can think about changing your lifestyle. Deep down inside though you know that the quick fixes are only temporary. And you know that if you want to keep your weight under control the best and healthiest way to do it is by changing the way you eat, not for two weeks, but for every day of your life.

It may comfort you to know that you are not alone. Perhaps the reason we don't simply do what seems obvious and sensible--EAT LESS AND EXERCISE MORE-- is because it's just not as simple as it looks. Wearing a patch on your arm for 2 weeks to lose weight is easy. Skipping a meal is easier than counting calories. These are temporary solutions. Then when you gain the weight back (because you didn't change your lifestyle), you lament.

Getting your weight under control is a primary step towards good health and improved self-esteem. Cosmetic reasons are not the only reasons to lose weight. More important is the benefit to your health.

Almost all of us have had the experience of not being healthy and often when we have recovered from our illness, we soon forget our misery. For many chronic diseases we feel just a little bit not well. It depends on the day or our mood. We just are not sick enough to do anything about it. But a major event will get our attention. When a life threatening illness strikes (like a heart attack) as we are carted into the Intensive Care Unit we resolve that from this day forward we will change our lifestyle habits, turn over a new leaf, and live in a healthy way. After a close call we become thankful for every day and treasure what health remains.

Life threatening events and permanently disabling threats to our bodies have an "awakening" effect. You are never quite the same again and if fortunate, a lesson is learned, and you become a happier more thankful person who treasures what amounts to another chance. You become very motivated to change habits to preserve your health.

As an epidemiologist I learned that interventions can be implemented at very different levels often with the same result. For example, both the wearing of seat belts and driving at a reduced 55 miles per hour speed limit do save lives on the highway. The interventions are different, but each action works to reduce the highway death toll: one by reducing driver impact inside the car, and the other by reducing the number of automobile accidents in the first place.

From psychology I learned that emotional factors can override a person's own best interest. Self-sabotage and bad habits keep many of us from enjoying optimal health and

12

happiness. And from nutrition I learned that there is much art to the science of eating. We are all specialized chemistry sets and what we eat sets the wheels in motion and keeps them going, but genetics play an important role as well.

My experience in the health field has taught me that perhaps one of the most debilitating factors in the lives of most mobile "healthy" people is simply being overweight. In general it does not contribute to people's happiness and almost always it will accelerate any predisposing physical condition and make treatment for any medical problems more difficult.

If there was one public health intervention I could recommend that would reduce premature death, physical ailments, surgery and its complications, and reduce the risk of most chronic diseases it would be for all people to eat properly, exercise moderately, and keep their weight in a healthy range. ***That's why I wrote this book.*** If we could all do this, fewer hospitals would be built and our health costs would nose-dive. We would all be healthier and happier people.

Most articles and books that are written by those trained in nutrition are based on sensible eating principles and focus on the ability of foods to meet nutritional needs as opposed to weight loss needs. However, when nutritionists do create reduced calorie diets for weight loss they can become very complicated because there is tremendous focus on getting the right daily nutrients into the body. Therefore food tables are needed so that nutritionally similar foods can be grouped and interchanged with one another. The quantities must be limited and from a dietician's exacting point of view, they should be weighed or measured so that portions are comparable. Almost all well-balanced diets for weight loss include exchange tables, food groups, and measured quantities of food as caloric and/or nutritional equivalents. Sometimes these requirements are met in a liquid or powdered form. However, the best diets use real foods that you can buy in the supermarket.

Attempting to fill the gap are many commercial programs to help people lose and maintain their weight loss. I spoke with one graduate of such a program. She exclaimed how she lost 12 pounds on this nationally advertised program. I asked her if she now knew how to eat and she said, "Yes." What she learned was to eliminate almost all fat from her diet and to eat a diet containing very specific percentages of protein and carbohydrate. This program sold pre-packaged food which adhered to these stipulations. While she was in the program she simply ate the pre-packaged dinners. She did not die, but she was very hungry and her hair started to fall out. She was now on what she called "maintenance". She ate an orange and a banana for breakfast, a salad from a local salad bar for lunch with no butter or oil and for dinner she had a small portion of meat and a salad and a plain roll. Of course, she mentioned it was difficult for her to eat that way all the time, but she was trying. I told her she was on a "deprivation diet" and that it was quite understandable that she would be hungry. What she had learned from this program was to eliminate fat from her diet and to cut down on her portions. All very well and good, as long as she bought the pre-packaged meals. However, she still didn't know how to eat. And for maintaining weight loss on your own, you need to know how to eat. My prediction sadly is that she will eventually gain back all the weight that she lost. I am reminded of that Chinese proverb that states: "*If you give a man a fish you feed him*

dr. Anne plan

for a day. If you teach a man to fish you feed him for a lifetime". In a sea of so many diet alternatives consumers are confused and want to believe that they will be successful with the doctor who prescribes pills or liposuction, the nutritionist who offers laborious recipes for reduced calorie menus or the packaged program "consultant" who advertises quick results with celebrity endorsement. All of these programs will work for a time. Unless you can maintain the weight loss on your own, however, you will continue to bounce from one weight loss scheme to another.

The healthiest way to lose weight is through exercising and living a well-balanced eating lifestyle. In this book you will soon have the tool for staying healthy and staying slim. You are invited to learn a way of living and eating that can stay with you for all time.

Finding the 'magic' of a simple solution
After studying many nutritionally sound diets, I was able to distill the well-balanced, but often complicated guidelines into one easy system. What makes our MagicHand apprach easy is that you do not need to count calories or weigh foods in order to eat nutritiously and to have a well-balanced diet. I reasoned that If I could find a way to make nutritious well-balanced eating easy and exercise enjoyable, perhaps more people would do it.

From the starting chapter in this book you will learn how to eat. The unique feature, and the basic tenet of the entire eating plan, is to use the hand to measure portion sizes. This does not mean you scoop rice into your hand! But, some foods like an apple, you can hold. The hand becomes a visual estimator and measuring tool. This is what eliminates counting calories and using exchange tables. This is what separates MagicHand eating from all other programs making it a cinch to use. But, there's much more to it than that-- you can eat what you want, when you want, and what everyone else is eating. You will learn to eat the way a person eats who wants to stay slim without the feeling of being deprived. If you must, you could even eat French fries (although I'd hope for a better choice).

Weight loss is gradual and natural, averaging 1 to 2 pounds a week. You may lose more or less weight than that in a week depending on how overweight you are at the onset and on how grudgingly your body insists on holding on to fat. However, most people will reach their ideal weight within six months. If you need only to lose a few pounds it could happen in a month. Thereafter the weight loss is maintained forever by continuing to follow the MagicHand guidelines. It becomes a way of life for those who want to stay slim. And, like magic, the pounds vanish.

What you will learn is how to eat with a few simple hand tricks. The precise performance of these hand maneuvers will bring about the desired weight control outcome. And you will know what to eat. Each Point in this book focuses on an aspect of health that will help you maintain your ideal body weight. The eating plan itself is easy to follow and implement, but you will need to integrate exercise into your life as well. I believe that sharing with others helps to keep us motivated and I suggest that after you read each Manual chapter that you complete the corresponding Practice Point section.

You may already have many good habits in place. For example, some people already reserve time for meditation whereas others say they have no time. Read each Point chapter, nine altogether, and decide if the subject applies to you. Regardless, answer the questions on the relevant Practice page. You will get the most from this book if you read every Point and complete each Practice Point.

MANUAL and PRACTICE: The Manual is in the front part of this book and contains the content-- what you need to know to follow the Plan. After you read the Point chapter, go to the Practice part of the book. Find the corresponding Point, and answer the questions for self-discovery and practical application. This Practice section addresses issues relevant to each Point. You can complete the questions by yourself or discuss your answers with others in a Practice Circle.

Practice Circle: We recommend at least three people to start a Practice Circle. (See Appendix C for details.) If you want to open your Circle to others, list your group on the internet and start a Zoom, Webex, GoogleMeet, Zoho, in-person or other type of meeting. Going through the Practice questions with others will help give you the support you need to live the program. After you finish all nine Points, repeat the Points again and again. You will find that each time you repeat the process you will learn something new about yourself. Being with others lends support and keeps you motivated.

And to stay motivated at home repeat each Point-- read just two pages each day!

Look terrific. Feel great. That's the result.

APPORTION

Point 1: Measure
Point 2: Hold
Point 3: Adapt

● Point 1: Measure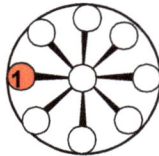

How to visualize portions

Even among well-educated Americans knowledge of how to lose weight properly is lacking. Whatever your profession or line of work, your concept of how to lose weight probably has been influenced by a barrage of television and print ads, magazine articles and podcasts, each claiming something special about a new product or finding. Separating the wheat from the chaff becomes a Herculean task. Perhaps underlying all of this is the fantasy or wish for a magic solution. We want to believe that with one pill, with one divine potion, our excess pounds will disappear! This is the fairy tale that we want to come true. When I wave the magic wand all your cellulite will disappear; the fat will dissolve and you will live happily ever after. Truth be told there is no <u>one</u> magic potion. But, there are rituals--lifestyle rituals-- that if followed will make it seem like magic. You can attain weight-loss by changing the way you literally look at food.

In my first healthy diet book (1982) I brought to national attention the concept of using your hand to visually measure food portions. Many other programs have adopted this idea since then but this program remains the first and only program relying completely on the hand for food measure. It is imprecise making it nutritionally variable. There's a trade-off I was willing to make between a program being livable or a program strictly following Recommended Daily Allowances (RDA). It also had to be flexible— adaptable to changes in Federal nutritional recommendations and adaptable to medically restricted diets. Olympic level top health is a great goal, but good health is more readily achieved. This program is every day livable! However, Practice remains key.

In this chapter you will learn how to use what Dr. Anne calls the MagicHand to gauge portion sizes for weight-loss and weight-control. It's a hand trick that works like "magic" to produce results. And your hand is with you wherever you go!

What you also will find in this chapter is actually a re-learning of what you probably already "know" and suspect is true: that eating regular balanced meals throughout your life is healthy, and the best way to permanent weight loss.

Nevertheless I can understand the desire to want to believe in fairy tales and quick solutions. I'll never forget the woman who came running over to me at one of my first MagicHand Eating Plan seminars. She was so excited and enthused about this new diet and asked, "Tell me, where is the spot that I press on my hand to lose weight?" She was educated, intelligent and "knew" better, but still wanted to dream that maybe this would be an instant solution; maybe this would be a trick that would work. Maybe this time she hoped she could just press the magic spot on her hand and lose ten pounds. Don't we all wish? It is difficult to face the pain and reality that being overweight means that we just ate too much or lacked exercise. Truly it is not the end of the world and wonderfully it is correctable through healthy balanced eating and moving your body.

You need not take drugs. You need not endure drastically invasive measures. The choices are clear: You must simply decide whether you want to engage in a yo-yo struggle of weight loss and weight gain, **OR** whether you want to invest in modifying your lifestyle by altering your eating habits. Both scenarios apply for a lifetime.

In the first situation your normal eating is a weight-gain diet and to lose the weight, it is corrected by sometimes severe and restrictive diets or fasting episodes. This cycle repeats itself.

In the second situation your normal weight-gain diet is corrected by balanced eating to maintain your desired weight. The cycle is broken; weight control is permanent. It is corrected by re-education and changing habits. It's YOUR choice.

In this book you will get the special knowledge you need to break that lifetime yo-yo cycle. Be assured that this program has been tested and that it is easy to follow and to live with for the rest of your life. Others have done it and you can too. Assuming you have decided that healthy weight loss is preferable to any other alternative, you have made the right choice.

How do we start? We start by recalling an earlier time when we were in grammar school and our teacher told us about proper eating and good nutritional habits. To gain back this fundamental knowledge that we may have lost over the years, a review of the basic nutritional concepts underpinning a well-balanced diet is required reading. In the pages ahead you will relearn what may seem quite elementary, but it is also important because it provides the foundation for balanced meal planning.

Your first homework assignment

I know that you're very anxious to get started on this program and to start losing weight right away. But if you really want to get maximum benefit and knowledge from this training, I'd like you to select three consecutive days of your life, and write down everything you eat, and the time of day. If you are involved in some physical exercise also include the activity and time of day. Be honest, after all this record is for your eyes only. This nutritional diary will establish your baseline and identify some of the foods you like to eat on a regular basis. As you learn how to use your MagicHand it will have more meaning to you and you will be better able to judge how to reconstruct your present way of eating.

You will need a sheet of paper for Day 1, Day 2 and Day 3. Or you can write directly in this book on the following table.

For three days, track these meals		
Day 1	Day 2	Day 3
BREAKFAST:		
LUNCH:		
DINNER:		
SNACKS:		
TOTAL CALORIES:_____		
ACTIVITIES? What did you do to "burn up" calories each day, for how long?		

18

If you can find the calories on the package of the food item you consumed, or you have an approximate idea or access to a calorie book, add the number of calories for each day.

This will be your "before the program" record-- and you can then compare that with how you now will be eating.

Basic training begins
Feel free to skip this section if you already know about food groups!
Go to the "Seeing Fingers" section in this chapter.

Do you remember the charts our teachers would display showing us the Basic Four Food Groups? These foods were considered essential for inclusion in our daily diet.

Pictured was a luscious carrot and robust head of cabbage, a container of milk behind a cut section of cheese, apples, oranges, and a well-done steak nested against a fresh water trout. These selected foods were representatives from the Basic Four Food Groups: (1) Fruits & Vegetables, (2) Milk & Dairy, (3) Meats, and (4) Bread & Cereals. The Basic Four Food Groups were established many years ago as a guide to insure adequate intake of many of the essential nutrients including proteins, vitamins, and minerals. The foods are grouped together on the basis of similarities in composition and nutritive value.   In theory if you ate foods every day from each of the groups you could be reasonably confident of eating a nutritionally adequate or balanced diet.

As youngsters we knew that in order to balance a diet, foods from these various food groups had to be included in our daily meals. But as adults many of us have forgotten the basics: in order to balance a diet, to make it nutritionally sound, we must eat from a variety of food groups. If a diet does not include foods from these various groups on a daily basis it is probably unbalanced, and that means unhealthy!

Your body demands a variety of foods--at least 44 essential nutrients--to adequately meet its needs for cell repair and function. That is why any diet proposing that you eat as much as you want of only one food is inherently dangerous. You may lose weight initially on a poor diet because psychologically you can only eat so many bananas or pineapples in one day. Eventually, however, your body "hungers" for what it needs and it is not unusual for people to gain all their weight back plus some after a deficient diet because now the body has experienced nutrient deprivation and reacts by "storing" energy to increase survival odds. Wouldn't you do the same thing?

If suddenly you no longer had all of the items you needed, you would make sure to get twice as much the next time. Many Americans are on chronic deprivation diets while their bodies are busy storing or adding fat. This doesn't make sense. The deprivation is nutritional but the body's compensation is caloric. The body reasons that if it eats enough food--whatever is available--it is more likely to find the missing nutrients. This may be a good strategy in the jungle. Translating to modern times this means that people who are on extremely low-calorie diets (less than 1,000 calories a day) are simply not meeting their needs for important nutrients and because of this severe deprivation they will later stock up with calories. I guarantee that if you eat well-balanced meals, not only will you look and feel better and lose weight, but you will be astonished by how <u>much</u> you can eat. And your body will not be signaling physiological nutritional hunger. If you experience hunger it is more likely to be of the psychological variety common in binge eaters (to be addressed later).

The habits we have formed as adults have contributed to whatever shape we now find ourselves. If you want to break the cycle of degenerative bad health and weight gain, then you must be willing to change your habits. Using the MagicHand you will quickly learn what food groups you tend to favor at the expense or exclusion of others. For example, Doreen, a bank employee loves donuts in the morning, eats a sandwich for lunch, and often a t.v. dinner (because she's too tired to cook) in the evening. This is a normal diet for many people, but UNBALANCED, UNHEALTHY. Doreen is overweight, and she doesn't eat much. Her problem is she doesn't eat correctly. If she balanced her food groups, she could eat even more and lose weight.

Federal guidelines in recent years expanded the number of Food Groups which is in accordance with what our Plan recommends. When eaten daily these foods will give you the balanced diet you deserve, and when carefully portioned you can be assured of healthy, permanent weight-loss.

The six MagicHand Food Groups are (1)Milk & Dairy, (2)Fruits, (3)Carbohydrates, (4)Protein, (5)Oils & Fats, and (6)Vegetables. You must know what foods fall into the various food groups to balance your diet. Most people know, for example, that an apple is a fruit--but how do you know if kidney beans are a carbohydrate or a protein? Sometimes a food can actually belong in more than one group. The kidney bean for example is considered an excellent source of protein (especially for vegetarians) and could substitute for meat or fish. It is also a complex carbohydrate, and could be used in meal planning as a substitute for bread, cereal or pasta.

According to nutritionists we need to eat foods from different food groups to keep our bodies building and repairing. For example, we need protein for tissue repair and we need carbohydrates or starches for quick energy. (The kidney bean does both!) We also need fat (although non-essential) which is easily found in butter and oil. Fat isn't <u>all bad</u>- it helps to store vitamins and to some degree protects our organs. I can hear you saying, "I don't need fat!"

Depending on what text you read the recommended food groups may vary in number, but all include fruits, vegetables, milk and dairy products, whole grains, and protein. The bottom line is that for your nutritional well-being, foods from each of these groups should be included in your daily menu.

To keep these food groups firmly in your mind what follows is a brief summary of the food groups included in our program and the nutrients they supply as well as other tidbits (pardon the pun) of information! Here is a brief review of our SIX FOOD GROUPS:

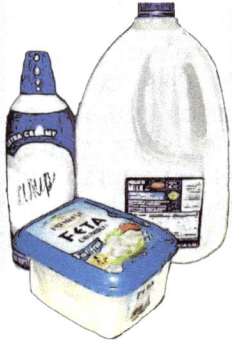

(1) MILK & DAIRY

Milk is generally considered an almost perfect food because it supplies protein for tissue building, calcium for bone growth, and riboflavin for the metabolism of amino acids. Dairy products most people are familiar with are buttermilk, yogurt, cheese, and yes, ice cream! Look for the low-fat cheese and milk products. It is a false saving if you are worried about calories and skip milk. In the portion sizes we recommend you will not gain weight and for women, especially over 40, calcium reserves are important in order to curtail bone loss and prevent osteoporosis.   While milk is considered by some to be an almost "perfect" food, it does not supply adequate amounts of Vitamin C. And that is why we need:

(2) FRUIT

Vitamin C is the only vitamin not stored in our bodies, so it must be constantly replenished.   Fruits also are wonderful for supplying roughage and keeping our sweet tooth in check. In fact this may be why we humans have a sweet tooth--so that we would eat fruit! Unfortunately many of us got carried away with sweets, and have been paying the price ever since. Although many nutritionists lump the vegetable and fruit food groups together since both are good sources of vitamin C, on our Plan we separate fruits and vegetables into different food groups. Fruits are usually quite different calorically from vegetables. You can get your sweet fix from an apple, or an orange, or a peach or some strawberries.

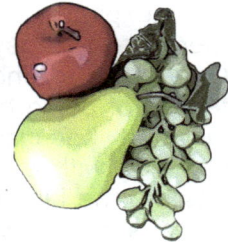

The next three food groups are labeled as Carbohydrate, Protein and Oil. Almost all foods contain some of each of these nutrients. Foods relatively high or considered a good quality source of that component are classified in that food group.

(3) CARBOHYDRATE

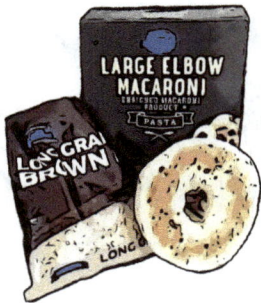

This food group includes grains, breads and cereal products as well as rice and pasta.   Besides supplying "quick energy", additional riboflavin, niacin and iron are gained from these foods. Of course, the more natural the product and the less refined, the more likely the food is to contain other trace vitamins and minerals as well. And the less refined the food, the more roughage also. We recommend complex carbohydrates for weight reduction over foods containing simple sugars. Potatoes and corn are also included in this category (rather than in vegetables) because of their high (complex) carbohydrate content. These complex carbohydrates when combined with legumes also supply quality protein.

(4) PROTEIN

When most people think of protein they think of meat, and many nutritionists feel that the "best" proteins are animal proteins because their essential amino acid composition is closest to that of human protein. It is also true that animal proteins generally contain

21

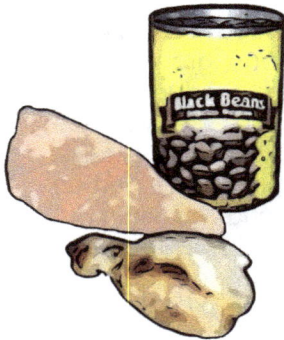

more fat than vegetable proteins so there is a trade-off. However, to utilize animal protein fully, plant protein is also necessary. For vegetarians, soybeans are considered a complete protein. To get a complete protein vegetarians can combine foods (like corn and beans) which can be consumed at the same meal or hours apart. Nevertheless getting enough Vitamin B-12 is in short supply in the vegetable world. For the B-complex vitamins the best sources are beef, pork, lamb, fish and poultry. Good quality protein is also found in eggs, nuts, lentils, dry beans, peas and legumes. We need protein for muscle and tissue building and repair.

(5) OILS AND FATS & sweets

There is one important reason for including oils and fats in your diet. Here experience has been my teacher. While you are losing weight there are two psychological saboteurs that can really get you down. One is the feeling of deprivation ("I can't have") and the other is the feeling of being hungry ("I want to eat all the time"). Oils and fats are included because usually people accustomed to butter will feel deprived without a pat of butter on their toast. But more importantly, fats are the last food to be digested in the stomach, so the feeling of being satisfied with your meal, with not being hungry, lasts longer when you include some fat at each meal. How much fat you should include will be discussed in the next section. Sweets and syrups also fall under this category in our program because while non-essential they are to be very limited.

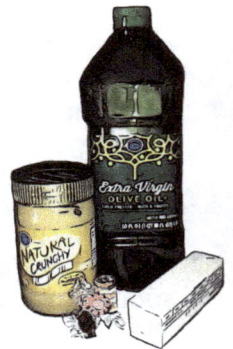

(6) VEGETABLES

On a plan to lose weight, vegetables are your best friends. They do so much and for so little. Not only do they provide vitamins and minerals and roughage, but they are filling, satisfying, tasty and contain hardly any calories! The Vegetable food group includes green ones like broccoli, spinach, and lettuce, and the so-called yellow ones like carrots and winter squash, rich in vitamin A.

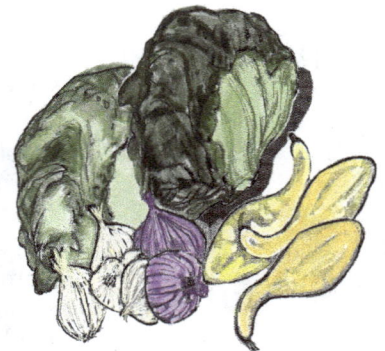

You will recognize that all well-balanced diets are basically the same. That's because they **are** including all the food groups nutrionists recommend.

To summarize, the food groups to be included in your daily eating are:
* Milk and dairy products
* Fruits
* Carbohydrates
* Proteins
* Oils & Fats
* Vegetables

It sounds like a lot of food, but just to meet your body's basic nutritional requirements about 1200 calories (of the "right" foods) would be minimal. Fewer calories than that could actually stress your body and contribute to nutritional deficiency. If you want to lose weight, changing the quality of your diet will help, but it is not enough. Portion size must be limited, and exercise increased. Of these six food groups, only one food group needs no restriction. Can you guess which one? Vegetables are so low in calories and so filling that you can eat as many as you'd like and still not gain weight. Remaining are five food groups requiring portion size restriction and these are called the FIVE FINGER FOOD GROUPS.

Again, altogether there are six food groups on the Plan and the FIVE FINGER FOODS are subject to portion control. Can you imagine eating all these foods every day? How healthy you will feel, how lightly you will run, how wonderful it could be.

Now you know what you should eat for a nutritionally sound balanced diet. But to lose weight the knowledge of "what" is not enough. You need to know "How much?" What follows is **some** magic-- some sleight of hand!

Your hand is the tool

If you are familiar with well balanced diet plans you are also familiar with the exchange tables used to help balance the diet. These exchanges are designed to work with the food groups to insure adequate amounts of required nutrients. For example, in a standard daily menu two servings of meat may be recommended. This will meet your daily requirement for protein. However, to know what is meant by a serving for each specific food (because not all foods, for example, will contain the same amount of protein) you must refer to a table listing exchanges. Using the Meat Food Group for protein, one serving of meat with 7 ounces of protein could be one lean frankfurter or one serving of meat could also be a one-ounce portion of fish both at about 45 calories. These two "meats" in these quantities are nutritional equivalents hence the use of the word exchange. Confusing on how to implement, yes.

While the system is excellent for people who have the time and energy to create menus using the lists, the system while technically suited for dietitians who meal plan, is just too complicated for most of us. Weighing foods is not for everyone. Yet I am a believer in the well-balanced diet, and I feel that the reason many people resort to "quick fixes" like liquid diets and unbalanced two-week wonder diets is because they need something easy, something that requires no thought, and/or something that they can just pour out of a box for a week.

The problem is that after that week is gone, most people return to their same eating pattern which is a weight-gain diet! How long will your weight loss last? And what will be your next diet? The next one may be harmful; the next one might even kill you. Because I believe so strongly in healthy weight-loss, the diet I developed had to be healthy. But it also had to be easy to follow and easy to remember and livable for a lifetime. And yet I promise-- you will not be deprived of your favorite foods. You will simply learn how to eat in a healthy way, eating regular meals, with portion sizes controlled. Unbelievable? You'll soon see that it works.

In order to make following a healthy well-balanced diet practical and easy I wanted to find a way of establishing a standard serving size that would work across all food groups. This would eliminate the use of scales for weighing foods, and reference tables. The tool that I realized way back in 1980 that is so practical and (literally) so handy to use is the hand. (And I wrote a book about it in 1982) The MagicHand was the original, the first weight loss diet plan to exclusively use the hand measure for portions. The idea really spread and I know that other programs have now incorporated this measure to varying degrees. The hand is the "natural" eating utensil of man; the tool we used before we invented the knife and fork. Our early forebears ate nuts, fruits and seeds from the palms of their hands.

The measurer is your own hand! But don't envision yourself dipping your hand into cooked foods. Your hand does not replace a knife and fork. All you really need in order to follow this program is various parts of your hand to **gauge portions**. You will learn to **visualize** the correct portion size. This requires **your** judgment. Food is handled only when it is natural to do so. (For example, holding an apple.) Your hand can also be placed over the food. (For example, in gauging the size of fish.) And you will keep track of your food groups by using your fingers to count the FIVE FINGER FOODS.

Using your own body part as a measurer has historical significance. The "hand" is a unit of length originally defined as the width of a man's hand from the little finger to the thumb.   Units of various lengths known as hand or palm were used by the ancient Egyptians, Hebrews, Greeks, Romans and others. Because there was no better way, people used parts of their bodies to measure things. The "palm" was the width of four fingers and a "yard" was the length from the end of your nose to the end of your hand. These measures were always available and easy to use. The inch was the length of a man's thumb joint. As the Romans marched all over Europe they left behind common units of length. With the ability to measure precisely, the hand became standardized at 4 inches (10.16 centimeters) from a statute decreed by Henry VIII of England. In the recipe for his Crepes Suzettes, Henri Charpentier, the cook for Albert, the Prince of Wales, describes placing the amount of butter in a skillet as one joint of your thumb.

Time honored "Units of Personal Measure" include the breadth of a thumb (1 inch), the flat palm, and the phalanx which is the terminal phalanx of the thumb. In a Farmstead magazine article David Tresemer describes how to plant a garden. He says that "carrots grow better at a phalanx apart than 2 inches apart". He claims that when you measure your garden this way you can perceive the garden as a measure of yourself. In similar fashion, when you use your own personal measuring stick, your own hand, you will feel more closely connected to your intake.

Moreover, the hand's breadth is a measure still used today to measure the height of horses from the ground to the withers. And your own hand is the tool we will use. (But you will not be eating like a horse!)

The hand is used as the measurer for portion or serving size. You literally have a helping hand. We can envision what would fit into our cupped hand or what would fit under the outline of the palm of our hand. Rather than to rely on a technical instrument to give us

24

a reading we can use one of our senses-- sight. We can look at a portion size and determine if it is the same size as a specific part of our hand. The advantage to this measuring tool over all others is that you always have it with you (convenience) and the size of your hand is naturally proportioned to your body and bone structure. Everyone has a different size hand and it is the right size for them! As you might expect, the smaller the person, the smaller the hand. We will use the hand as a measurer and as a reminder of what foods to include at each meal. It governs only the FIVE FINGER FOOD GROUPS that need to be controlled in order to achieve successful weight loss and management: (1) Milk, (2) Fruit, (3) Carbohydrate, (4) Protein, and (5) Fat.

So let's take a look at your hand. Focus on your palm and imagine that in the palm you could fit an apple, or a small roll or a hamburger patty. For example, my palm measures about 3" X 4" and when cupped would hold about one-third of a cup of something. These palm portion helpings are correct amounts to eat for losing weight and ironically in most cases are very close to the serving amount recommended on the "official" food group exchange tables. No calculating, no weighing foods: you can gauge portion size by just imagining what would fit in your own palm! Could it be any easier to correctly size a portion? The size of your own hand is very concrete, very exact, and not really subject to interpretation. Something either fits in your palm or it does not. (Loose interpretations are tantamount to cheating or taking extra amounts on this program.)

Seeing Fingers

Let's look at your hand again. We'll study the fingers this time. O.K., five on each hand. And five food groups that need monitoring. Again, they are: Milk, Fruit, Carbohydrate, Protein and Fat. So now you know that for cheese, fruit, cereals, breads and other baked goods, and meat, poultry and fish, and butter, fats and oils that it is the size of your own hand--palm and thumb--that governs the portion size.

If you will, please follow these instructions with me and actually do what I say. Remember you will be visualizing the foods that you eat in relationship to your hand size. When practical you can actually place the food in your hand.

Look at *your right hand with the palm facing you. Starting with your pinky assign a word to each finger. Your pinky is "My", the next finger is "Fingers", the middle finger is "Count", the index finger is "Portions" and the thumb is "Offering" (Variety). This phrase will help you to remember the food groups and the fact that their portion size is governed by your hand: Milk, Fruit, Carbohydrate, Protein, and Oils.*

You may have noticed that the first letter of each word in the phrase "**M**y **F**ingers **C**ount **P**ortions **O**ffering" corresponds to the first letters of the FIVE FINGER Foods. To remember the food groups:

My	**F**ingers	**C**ount	**P**ortions	**O**ffering	**V**ariety
Milk	Fruit	Carbohydrate	Protein	Oils	Vegetables

While you hold this book in your left hand look again at your right hand (with your palm facing you). As you can see there are four fingers directly above your palm. These four fingers represent the four food groups-- Milk, Fruit, Carbohydrate and Protein. Serving sizes for these are gauged using the palm of your hand. The food should fit within the parameters of your palm and you can either hold the food in your hand or visually match your palm to the food portion. The helpings are called palm portions.

The only finger we haven't discussed is your thumb representing the Oils food group. Look again at your hand. The serving size for Oils and Fats & Sweets is governed by your thumb joint size. You are "offered" a very small portion.

You may notice we did not include Vegetables as a food group monitored by the hand. And that is because you can eat as many vegetables as you please on this program. Portions are not controlled. But to remind yourself, look at your hand again and see that between the index finger and the thumb is an open "V", and that is for Vegetables! Memorize this slogan while studying your hand for the next three minutes. "**M**y **F**ingers **C**ount **P**ortions **O**ffering **V**ariety." Look at your fingers and that open "V". Say "My Fingers Count Portions Offering Variery" as you go from pinky to thumb. Offering what? "Variety".

Look at the fingers above the palm governing Milk, Fruit, Carbohydrate and Protein, and visualize a food item from each food group fitting into your palm. (In the Seeing Fingers Appendix E you will find a list of foods that fall under each Finger Food Group category.) Go to your refrigerator and look for foods you could actually pick up and hold in the palm of your hand. Notice how one egg seems to fit perfectly in the palm of your hand. (That would be 1 Protein.) Then look at your thumb and visualize an oil, for example, a pat of butter-- the size of the first joint of your thumb! When you can clearly visualize these portions then you will know the serving size of foods from each food group. You will never be in doubt as to how much food to put on your plate. Look at your palm, visualize the portion, and serve yourself. However, there are a few refinements you should know about. In actual practice the questions arise, "How thick should the portion be?" "How do I measure a liquid?" The portion should be no thicker than your thumb held sideways with the thumbnail facing you. (My thumb held sideways measures 3/4 in.)

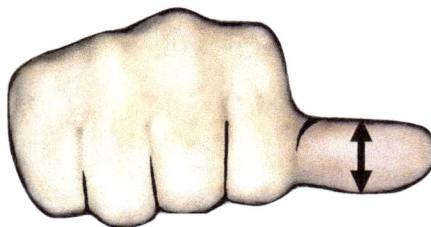

Some foods are better suited to sizing and visualization in a cupped palm. For example, a small tangerine would fit nicely in your cupped palm. If you could hold a liquid in your cupped palm about how much would it hold? Depending on your palm size it would be between 1/4 to 1/2 cup of liquid. That's the basic idea. Use your palm as a measurer for the four food groups represented by the fingers above the palm and, depending on the food, either cup the palm or use the hand's breadth and thumb thickness as a measure. Either hold the food in your hand or visually estimate the fit.

The Oils food group includes butter, margarine, mayonnaise and cooking and salad oils plus concentrated sweets. Because these foods are very high in calories the portion size is very small, no larger than your thumb to the knuckle joint. That means that on your palm size slice of bread (no thicker than your thumb) you could have a thumb knuckle's worth of butter!

The FIVE FINGER FOODs are controlled by the size of the palm and thumb of your own hand. You need never leave home without it! And once you actually practice this system it will be difficult to look at food servings any other way.

Food Groups

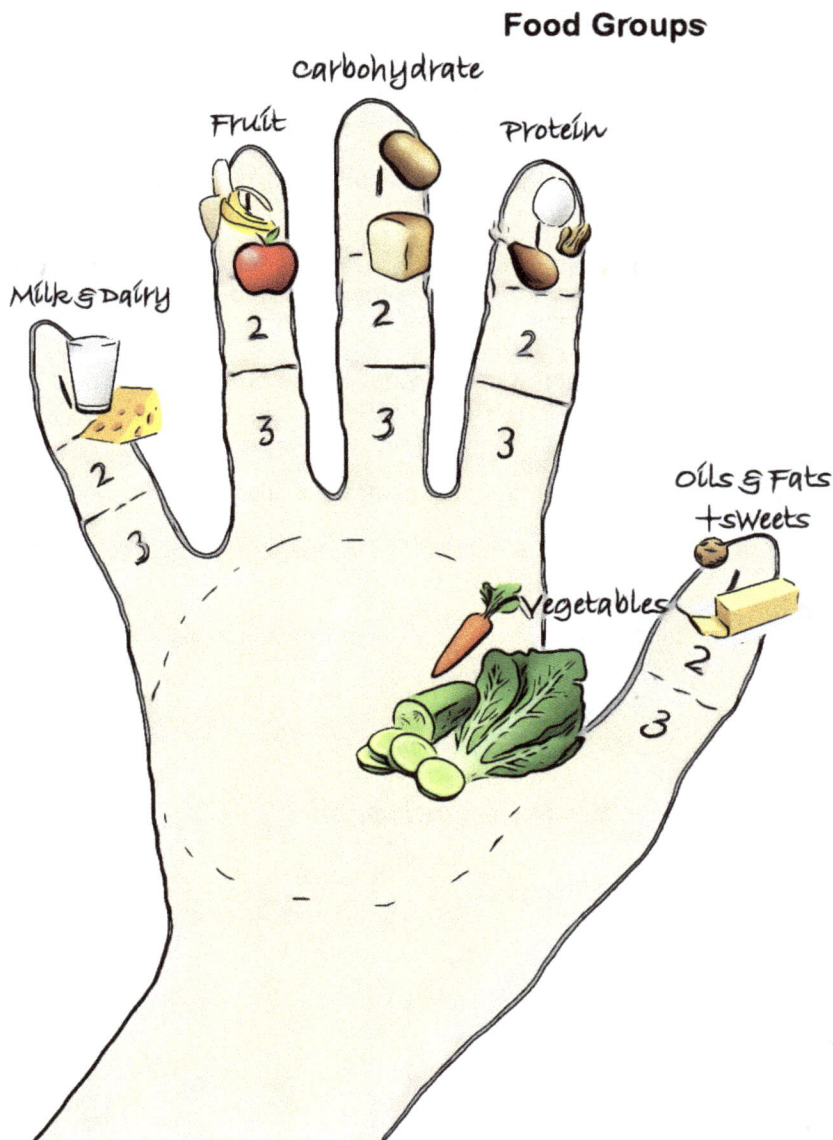

dr. Anne plan

Creating your MagicHand

It is now time for you to create your own MagicHand. This will be your own personalized hand to count portions.
You'll need a thick 8 1/2 X 11 sheet of paper, a pen, and five penny size magnets. And a surface for drawing.
(or copy the model on the facing page)

(1) **Write your first name** on the top.. Place your left hand palm down on the sheet of paper. Spread your fingers so there is enough room to trace between them. Now trace the outline of your hand using a pen.

(2) **Finger food groups**: Write above the pinky, Milk & Dairy; write above the thumb Oils & Fats; write above the middle finger Carbohydrates; write above the index finger Protein; write above the ring finger Fruit. In the open space between thumb and index finger, write Vegetables.

(3) **The palm**: Draw a light circle inside the palm of your hand. This is your personalized palm portion size.

(4) **Divide each finger into 3 joints** (to count the number of portions each day). You are permitted 3 palm portions for each food group above the palm and 3 thumbs for Oils & fats. All together you have 15 "chits": 12 palms and 3 thumbs!

(5) **Place the drawing** on your refrigerator with 5 magnets in the center of the palm. Every time you eat move the corresponding food group magnet to count the portion.

(7) **Count:** After you have moved the magnet 3 times for each food group, you have used all of your allotted chits for that day. (Remember, Vegetables are unlimited.)

(8) **Laminate** your drawing if you want to keep it in place for the rest of your life!

Your MagicHand!

(Your name)_____'s ***MagicHand***

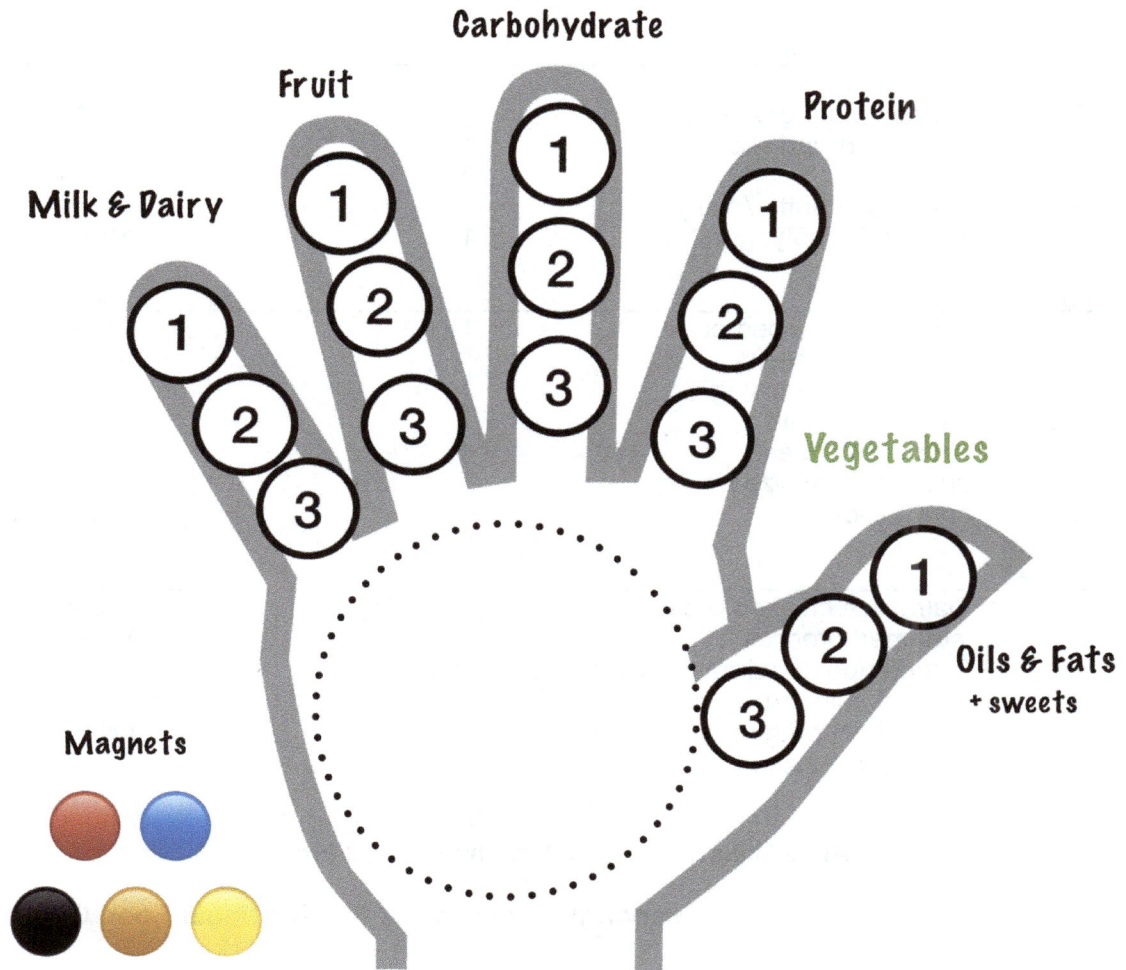

Carbohydrate

Fruit

Protein

Milk & Dairy

Vegetables

Oils & Fats
+ sweets

Magnets

How you want to distribute these servings over the day is your choice. In this way you could arrange to have a mid-morning and mid-afternoon snack. Here is a sample menu of what one day on the dr.Anne plan could include:

Meal	Quantity	Food Group
Breakfast		
1 cupped palm grapefruit	1	Fruit
1 palmsize bread slice	1	Carbohydrate
1 egg	1	Protein
1 thumb joint butter/marg.	1	Oil
Snack: 1/4 cup yogurt	1	Milk
Lunch		
2T. tuna fish/cupped palm	1	Protein
plate salad greens		Vegetable
1 thumb joint dressing	1	Oil
1 palm size bread	1	Carbohydrate
1 palm size cheese	1	Milk
Snack: 1 cupped palm size apple,	1	Fruit
carrot sticks		Vegetable
Dinner		
1 palm size chicken breast	1	Protein
steamed broccoli		Vegetable
1/2 cup(cupped palm). cream soup	1	Milk
1 cupped palm brown rice	1	Carbohydrate
1 thumb joint butter/marg.	1	Oil
1 sliced palm size peach	1	Fruit

TOTAL: 3 Milks, 3 Fruits, 3 Carbohydrates, 3 Proteins, 3 Oils

15 MagicHand servings: 3 servings from each of the five finger Food Groups.

plus unlimited Vegetables

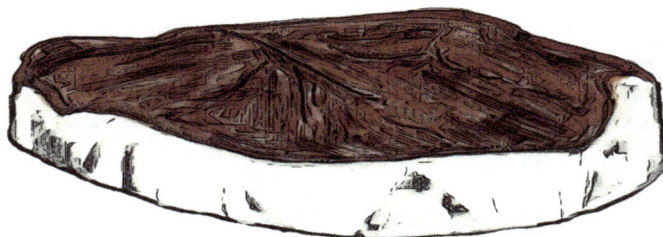

A portion that would fit in the palm of your hand!

Review the above portions on this menu and imagine these quantities fitting into your hand. Some you could actually hold in your hand and others would be gauged by holding your hand near the food. As you review the example given, move the magnets along your MagicHand drawing to correspond to the foods that are eaten for breakfast, lunch and dinner. You will have one magnet for each finger or each food group. Go through your meals, moving each magnet until all five magnets reach the number 3. This means you are through with the day's allotment of food. The next day you start all over again with all the magnets in the circle of the palm of the hand.

This is the technique you will use with your personalized MagicHand to lose weight and keep it off. Let's call the palm and thumb portions, chits. In this sense a chit is a voucher for a food portion. Think of it this way: you have a total of 15 chits a day-- 12 palm portions and 3 thumb portions. The palm portions can be flat and no thicker than your thumb, or rounded and visually fit in the palm of your hand. If you are in doubt, use a "palm-measure cap" from a coffee jar or something like that-- about 3/4 in. thick.

The thumb portions can be solid or liquid oils and visually be the size of your thumb. Milk, Fruit, Carbohydrate and Protein Food Groups are always in palm portions. Oils and fats are always in thumb portions. Vegetables are always as much as you want. Got it? Imagine that you are locked inside a room, and that you are only given 15 chits a day for your meals. How will you spend them?

Now imagine making your own menu including the foods from each food group that you like to eat. In the Practice section for this Point 1 you can create your own menus and list the foods you like under each Food Group. Remember there is no portion limitation for the Vegetable Food Group. On this Plan you will lose weight, preferably at a rate of 1 to 2 pounds a week, but if you are more than ten pounds overweight you can expect to lose even more every week.

Once you have reached your ideal weight (discussed in Point 4), then you can maintain that weight forever following this program, but perhaps not as strictly. Your MagicHand will always remind you of the food groups: the four food groups governed by palm portions, and the one food group governed by your thumb.

dr. Anne plan
The Golden Mean
In nature rainfall occurs at uneven intervals. One month's rainfall may be quite different from the next month's. Yet, on average, regions of the country are able to establish a general rainfall pattern for the year. Mother Nature tends to supply what is needed but She does so without concern for equally spaced or parceled rainfall. Mother Nature relies on the law of averages to keep this planet going. So, even if in one year the rainfall is below average, the next year might bring floods. In much the same way, the animal kingdom also survives. Sometimes feast, sometimes famine, but, on average, there is enough food to at least mature and produce a next generation. Fortunately we humans have greater control over our environment and do not need to suffer those extremes.

Nevertheless to meet our bodies nutritional requirements we do rely on the law of averages. We store many of the nutrients we need for healthy functioning in our cells, in our blood, and in our organs. Foods supply what we need, but not consistently, and depending on what stresses we encounter not always in the correct amount. However, on average, we are getting what we need from our foods to keep ready reserves and function well on a daily basis.

Please know that your body stores most vitamins & minerals-- and if needed supplies them on demand. As a safety net so that your stores of vitamin & minerals are adequate, I consider a daily multivitamin & mineral supplement that follows RDA (Recommended Daily Allowance) guidelines beneficial. However, high-doses of vitamins or minerals can create imbalances, become toxic, and I advise against that-- unless there is a clear deficiency, not responding to RDA, that diet can't correct.

Stretching this concept to an eating plan designed to lose weight and maintain weight loss, I believe we need not demand that every day's caloric intake be exactly the same. Following the laws of nature, some days would be different than others; some days may actually require more calories, and some days less calories. Typically a person's caloric intake and caloric expenditure actually tend to be very consistent. I am often impressed by the consistency with which many people keep their weight. Some people are "always" ten pounds overweight. And some people are "always" fighting five pounds. Mechanisms in our brain that control appetite are sometimes "set" at a weight other than the weight we want or the weight that might be healthiest for us. These mechanisms must be "re-set" and eventually through training and practice, we educate our bodies, but not always. For some people the only way weight loss can be maintained is to become conscious of foods consumed.

This Plan was designed to allow free choice of foods in all food groups. Certainly the foods in each food group are not exactly the same, neither nutritionally nor calorically. However, most of the foods in a food group do supply common nutrients. Where these foods can differ more significantly is in caloric value. With your MagicHand you do not keep track of calories. The emphasis is on portion control and not calorie counting. As in nature the law of averages becomes operative. When you use palm portions and vary your diet you will be eating different foods, some with more calories than others. Not all fruits, for example, are equal in calories even though they would fit in the palm of your hand. For example, a palm full of strawberries would have fewer calories than a palm full of grapes. The rule to be followed (if you are calorie-conscious) is that each palm portion should be approximately 100 calories. Usually this upper limit is automatically controlled by the palm portion size or will eventually average to 100 calories or less, so there is no reason to count calories. Just for your information, in the example I gave of strawberries and grapes, a half-cup of strawberries would be 29 calories and a half-cup of grapes would be 51 calories-- both well under 100 calories. The four food groups above the palm are 4 calories/gram and the thumb food group is 9 calories/gram. Weight of the food is the measure for most food-based programs. MagicHand is the one weight control program that relies only on hand volume as the measure.

The important tenet to remember is not how many calories you are eating, but whether the portion fits in the palm of your hand. This is the only rule you need to follow. Do not worry about the calories!

In our evaluations of caloric intake using our Plan the average daily intake varied between 1200-1500 calories a day depending on individual palm size and food selection. This is an excellent level of caloric intake for gradual weight loss. Very low calorie intake (less than 1000 calories a day) will result in weight loss, but generally for the short-term. No one can maintain that type of eating for very long, so most of these dieters gain all the weight back plus some to make up for the feeling of deprivation.

Foods differ and for this reason it is important to include a variety of foods in your diet. You can freely choose whatever foods you want to eat as long as they are palm portions. However, some foods are more "calorie dense" than nutrient dense, and that means more calorie-packed.

This is where the term empty calories applies: lots of calories and few nutrients. If, for example, you are counting a Brownie (palm-portion) as 1 Carbohydrate, that food is certainly higher in calories than a cupped palm of brown rice, which is also counted as 1 Carbohydrate. And I do not expect you to hold the cooked rice in your hand-- just visualize the portion! Calorie dense means that the food is rich, caloric, and probably looks thick and feels heavy. Most refined foods are very calorie dense (with low nutrient density). For losing weight quickly we recommend that you avoid the "calorie dense" foods, even if they fit in the palm of your hand. But when you have reached your goal weight then you can begin to include more "calorie dense" foods if you wish, still fitting in the palm of your hand, without going off this Plan. Nutrient dense foods, however, are much preferred and healthier. In general if you avoid the foods that contain high concentrations of any refined sugars you will be eating less calorie dense, more natural foods. For faster weight loss stay strictly with nutrient dense foods. However, if the situation arises where this is unavoidable or you simply "must" have some very calorie dense food, rather than to feel deprived, I recommend that you have a palm portion and satisfy your psychological hunger. You will still lose weight because you are using your MagicHand and the law of averages will eventually work. If sometimes you eat foods that are calorie dense and at other times you eat foods that are less dense, eventually the lower calorie foods will compensate for the higher calorie foods, and on average, you will be holding a steady weight-loss course. However, if you want to lose weight quickly, do not take too many detours!

As you practice eating this way you may have questions and as you continue to read the sections ahead hopefully they will be answered. You will learn the nuances and fine tune your eating-- finding your own way of living and your own food preferences.

Knowledge without action however is to no avail. In your heart you may feel that you "know" all of this is correct procedure and in fact, it couldn't be easier. But, there are saboteurs. Knowing what to do and actually doing it are two different things. The challenge is to make this way of eating a part of your life-- a way of eating that is so automatic that you notice the difference when you <u>don't</u> follow this Plan.

Over the years as I have taught seminars and workshops I have watched people lose weight and gain their own self-respect from achieving their goals. While the treatment I advocate may seem simple, the problem is complicated and deadly serious. Anyone who has struggled with being overweight knows that what I have presented so far is only one part of the picture.

This core of knowledge, however, of what and how to eat, is what needs to be learned and practiced over and over again to effect a lasting change. After all, what is magic but the precise performance of prescribed actions followed by specific outcomes: use the Magic of your own Hand for weight control.

To understand these measures in standard equivalents
See Appendix A.
To see what foods are in different food groups
See Appendix E.

Take away message: Control food intake using palm and thumb portioning. You can correct and change eating habits— you now know how to eat for the rest of your life.

● Point 2: Hold

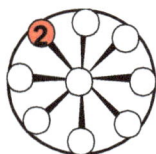

The definition of a chit
We identify palm portions and thumb portions as "chits". You can count "chits" as vouchers or tokens. For an entire day you get 12 palm size chits and 3 thumb size chits. A total of 15 chits each day.

These chits act as "advances" towards your eating budget. Again, you have 15 chits for the day: use them wisely. Use 3 chits and you have 12 left. AFTER you have reached your goal weight your MagicHand chits allotment for the day can become more flexible by making food group trades. For example, you could trade a Milk & Dairy chit to get an extra Protein chit. The objective here is to maintain your success, to *hold* your ideal weight.

Yes, you can eat cake
Are you destined for a life of food group monitoring and palm portion counting?   The answer is yes and no. The purpose of this Plan is to teach you how to function like a normally eating person who eats well, but does not gain weight. Since your hand is always with you and you now have been taught how to eat "with your eyes" you can go anywhere and use your MagicHand. The system is extremely adaptable to all situations, but you must learn how to use it so that you can live this way and not feel deprived. After you have reached your ideal weight, the challenge facing you is to maintain that weight, that dress or suit size, that wonderful feeling of being light for the rest of your life. While you were losing weight it was necessary to stay strictly with the assigned food groups and portion sizes in order to lose weight. The difference between losing weight and maintaining weight is that when you are losing weight you <u>must</u> choose healthy fiber-rich foods to fit into those palm portions. For example, your Fruit must be an apple, not a fruitcake! But when you are on maintenance, **after you have reached your ideal weight** and are staying within your ideal weight range, you can opt for more calorie-dense choices-- but still in palm portions! It is also possible, when you are maintaining to adhere strictly to the program for (let's say) five days of the week, but not on week-ends. You will always stay in the program, but through trial and error you will discover how much lee-way you can take. You will also want to maintain your health so do not stray too far, or take too many liberties from the original plan. Otherwise, you'll be back, sadly, where you started.

Maintaining-- the tricky part
Certainly you can grit your teeth, eat a healthy diet for nine weeks, lose weight, and consider your diet a success. But, the really tricky part, the part that separates the men from the boys, the women from the girls, is **maintaining** that weight loss. In the same breath may I say, that the best part of controlling your weight is not only reaching your goal, but staying there. Once you have reached your ideal weight, you can start to take some "liberties" with meal planning. Your favorite (calorie-dense) foods can creep back on the menu, but only occasionally, and in moderation. You will not have to live without French fried potatoes for the rest of your life! If you see that you are gaining weight again as you add back some calorie-laden foods, and you reach the upper limit of your

warning zone, that is the time to get right back on your strict MagicHand eating. I warn you-- do not deviate too much! The most important rule here is never to go two pounds over your ideal weight. (By the same token, don't allow yourself to go two pounds below your ideal weight either.) A two pound weight gain over your ideal weight is a clear warning that you **MUST** limit or restrict your intake again. Avoid the calorie-dense foods. If controlling our weight came naturally, we could allow free rein. The simple fact is that we-- who want to keep our weight under control-- will be governed by palm portions for the rest of our lives. As a result we will probably be eating healthier foods and living longer than others. A good deal!

Stretching palm portions
Most people enjoy eating an elegant and tasty dessert. I have discovered that everything is in "presentation". Often what separates a high-priced restaurant from the ordinary is the garnish on the plate! Just to give you an idea, here's a suggestion for how you could serve an orange as a sumptuous dessert at home. Take about six orange sections and place them in a dish, arranged like the petals of a flower with ends meeting in the middle. Put a few raisins in the center. Then sprinkle lightly with cinnamon and unsweetened cocoa. Eat with a small fork (and accompanying candlelight). You now have a beautiful dessert-- and it can be counted as 1 Fruit chit.

Another way to stretch your palm portions is to add fruit to whatever you ordinarily might have for dessert. For example, ice cream is a favorite at our house. What I do is take a half-palm of fruit, like blueberries, and a half-palm size (about 1 rounded tablespoon) of ice cream and put them both in a dish. I can still count this dessert as one palm portion, and I feel like I've had a bowl of ice cream, yet I've saved a lot of calories.

If you are someone who likes to indulge in potato chips or tortilla chips, here's a test of your self-discipline. These are high-fat, high calorie foods, so I don't recommend you eat them on a regular basis, but since you're human you just may get the urge. Take a paper towel and place it in front of you. Put your hand in the bag and fill your hand with as many potato or corn chips as you can hold. Place this palm full on the paper towel and carry it away. (Put the bag back in a cupboard where you can't see it.) That will be 1 palm portion of a Carbohydrate.

How can you count alcoholic beverages? Imagine the liquid fitting in the palm of your cupped hand. It would be between 1/4 to 1/2 cup or about 4-6 ounces. Your judgment and ability to visualize the liquid will enable you to determine the liquid palm portion. What I do to stretch my palm portion of an alcoholic beverage is to add water. It's sacrilege to Americans, but addng water to wine is not an uncommon practice in other cultures.

If you enjoy a before-dinner cocktail, how about some vegetable juice on ice with a slice of lemon? It's filling, and doesn't cost one chit. Healthy too.

Do you like hot cocoa? I do. I had to discover a way to stretch my palm portion of milk. I use 1 palm portion of milk (about 1/4 cup), 1 teaspoon of coffee, 1 tablespoon of cocoa powder, and fill my cup with hot water. Then I add a dash of cinnamon (or vanilla) and I enjoy my cup of hot chocolate.

What about pasta? Do you just love to eat pasta? I do. I am an original spaghetti kid. As a child my mother had difficulty getting me to eat anything else. And it continues to be one of my favorite foods. To me a plate full of spaghetti is a good dinner. The way I stretch my pasta is to take a palm full of pasta (about one ounce- you can weigh it dry), cook it, and then add it to a half bag of cooked frozen string beans or broccoli. On top I add tomato sauce made from tomatoes (no oil) with onions and garlic. I serve with a palm portion of parmesan cheese and I've only used 2 chits, 1 Carbohydrate and 1 Milk. If I add a palm portion of ground turkey to my sauce I will use another chit for Protein. I have what looks like a full plate of pasta and indeed I have fooled myself. After eating, I feel full and satisfied. See *Appendix B* for some recipes.

With casseroles, especially you will find, that you have no idea what foods are buried inside. The best thing to do is not to attempt food group dissection. Trade in a palm portion chit from one of your food groups and serve yourself a palm portion size of whatever it is, and count it as one chit.

You soon discover what food group foods you favor over others. One of my clients told me that her Fruit and Carbohydrate chits always are used first and then she has a hard time getting any Milk products into her diet. If you have plenty of Milk chits remaining, you could use one of those chits for that palm portion of casserole. You can trade. Just remember that the farther away you get from balancing different food groups, the less healthy is your eating. This Plan makes you very conscious of what you're eating and how much you're eating. Remember that you only make trades when you are on maintenance. If you notice any physical change or weight gain, nip it in the bud. You will be amazed at how quickly you can get back to your ideal target. Stay in control. You will discover the joy of maintaining the right weight for your body design and the satisfaction of well-balanced meals.

Juggling chits
We are using the word 'chit' to mean one palm portion or thumb serving from a food group. Each day you start with 15 chits (12 palm-portions and 3 thumb-portions). Since this is a forever eating plan, I recognize that you may want to eat more of one food than another at certain times, deviating from a strict adherence to our guidelines. That's O.K. as long as you trade in your chits from another food group. Let's say that my mother bakes my favorite bread for me and delivers the loaf to my door. Also, let's say it's a trigger food for me. One palm portion slice won't be enough. I want the whole loaf! Because I have **some** control over my eating, I could trade in my chits from other food groups so that I could have more of the bread. This makes me feel that I will not be depriving myself and that I can have as much as I want as long as I do so in palm portion sizes and with whatever chits I have remaining. The price I pay is not to have a very well balanced meal plan that day. It's a small price to pay in my opinion for my mother's home baked bread. This is why I am able and you will be able to control your eating using your MagicHand forever. On maintenance you **can** trade in chits from one food group to another.

Again, to **lose** the weight you must strictly follow the MagicHand and not trade food groups. When you are maintaining or want to **hold** your weight at the present level you can make trades (without gaining weight). To hold your weight you can be more flexible with food groups, but you must still keep counting thumb and palm-portions.

For people who are on special diets this is a particularly valuable feature of the eating plan. If you are a strict vegetarian you might want to trade in all of your Milk chits for Fruit chits. (You can meet your calcium requirement by eating healthy servings of broccoli and other greens.) Your Protein chits could be used for nuts or grains. You can use the food group chits to complement and balance your proteins, for example, having a palm portion of rice (Carbohydrate) with a palm-portion of kidney beans (Protein).

Mainly you need to be aware that, in general, whenever you make a trade, while you may be increasing the "livability" of the eating plan, you are also reducing its health quotient. I call this controlled cheating. If you are a binge eater still struggling to overcome the psychological components of your bingeing, binge in palm portions not to exceed the allowable limit. This will help you to exercise some control over your compulsion. The next day you might feel sick, but you won't feel as if you "lost it" totally.

Believe me I am not endorsing the behavior, but healing takes time, and regressions are to be expected. If you are trading chits, a good guideline to remember is that one chit should not exceed 100 calories. If you are not trading chits, don't concern yourself with the calories.

Juggling chits is not advised while you are trying to lose weight since it will slow down the weight-loss process. However, being out of control and returning to overweight is worse.

You may choose on some days not to count your chits. Decide beforehand what occasions these will be and allocate no more than nine days a year. For example, I never count chits on Thanksgiving Day. This does not mean that I go crazy with my eating, but I do eat more. This lets me know that my natural inclinations, left unchecked, are still to gobble! If I ate all that I wanted every day then I wouldn't look the way I want to look. If I want to look slim and feel good, then I have to eat less than I want to eat. It's as simple as that. I am a person who understands this problem. I know what it's like to struggle to keep your weight under control. I am sharing my success with you, and I continue to live what I preach. The truth may be that many of us have a genetic propensity to accumulate fat. Recognizing this fact, we work with what we are given. And we do what we must to counteract this beneficial survival trait while preserving our health for today's world.

Your vote
Some may be wondering why I haven't said not to eat eggs or butter or why I don't seem overly concerned with the specific foods you may choose under each food category. Certainly I am aware that some food elements are linked to disease, but I am also aware that it is a complicated issue. For example if you're worried about cholesterol, It depends on the type, and even if you get rid of all the cholesterol in your diet, the liver will manufacture its own. Similarly with salt and blood pressure. Only some people with high blood pressure will get a benefit from reducing the salt in their diet. And the science changes. One egg that fits in the palm of your hand is 1 Protein as far as I'm concerned,

and it's one of the best foods you can eat-- an excellent source of vitamins and minerals. Equally important as **what** you eat is to keep your weight under control. Excess body weight is in general devastating to good health and tends to exacerbate any underlying conditions you may have.

If you are concerned about your fat intake, I do not discriminate between margarine and butter. With three thumb joint portions a day you will not be eating too much! However not all fats are equal. Highly monounsaturated oils such as olive oil, canola and nut oils are believed to contribute to your health. Animal fats and other saturated fats are to avoided. More and more research seems to point in the direction that genetic disposition might be more in play than diet. You be the judge of what foods you want to include. I am also not going to persuade you to choose foods that are labeled as "low-fat" or as "low cholesterol". If you enjoy the food, if you like the taste, then eat it. It still counts as a 1 chit portion when you use your MagicHand since we don't count calories. Your one-calorie salad dressing is still a 1 thumb joint portion chit. I find that I buy both reduced calorie dressings and other richer dressings, using them both, depending on my mood and desire. I don't worry about gaining weight in either case, since my portions are under control.

While maintaining your ideal weight I would like to persuade you to continue to make healthy food choices. Fresh fruits, fresh vegetables, low-fat or non-animal origin proteins, low-fat milks and cheeses and complex carbohydrates are the best. Educate yourself and please your palate. You are the only person who knows what makes you feel good and healthy.

When I see people substituting some chemical substance for a real egg or using an artificial sweetener I think they may be misguided. These actions do not constitute a healthy lifestyle and are token attempts towards better health. Stay with the real foods, limit your intake, exercise regularly and reduce your stress-- that's the best ticket.

Whether you agree with my philosophy or not, you are free to choose the foods you want to include (even if you insist on chemical eggs). We all make our own choices and your judgment may be different than mine, and your doctor may recommend that you eat specific commercially prepared substitutes. I will not argue. Whatever foods you choose, **IF** you follow the Plan, you will lose weight and be able to keep your weight under control. Either way, the program works.

Sweet so-long
There *is* one food that I believe has no value in your diet. That is sugar also known as sucrose, dextrose, and corn syrup. Sucrose is not metabolized in the body the same way as starch and other complex carbohydrates. Sugars occurring naturally in fruits and vegetables can be handled by the body quite easily whereas refined concentrated sugar can aggravate sensitive pancreatic excretions. The body breaks down white sugar (sucrose) into glucose-- the end product of all the carbohydrate products we eat. When we eat large quantities of sugar, insulin from the islets of Langerhans in the pancreas is secreted into the bloodstream. If the pancreas is overstimulated too much insulin may be secreted. When this happens, the blood sugar level will fall and remain low, possibly causing a craving for more sugar. When people get crotchety or irritated sometimes it's

because their blood sugar level is low. People with hypoglycemia are especially prone to feeling hungry all the time and to becoming easily annoyed at the slightest provocation. Like drug addicts they need a sugar fix. And like drug addicts, the cure is to get unhooked from sugar.

The liver plays a vital function in controlling the normal blood sugar level by removing sugar from and adding sugar to the blood. The activity of the liver is controlled by hormones from the pancreas and adrenal glands. When the adrenal glands are stimulated during periods of strong emotional stress blood sugar levels increase and the result may be hyperglycemia (high blood sugar). When the pancreas can no longer provide insulin, the result is diabetes.

Our body was never designed to handle concentrated forms of sugar. Basically our body has no need for sucrose. When sugar intake exceeds the body's immediate needs, it is quickly converted to fat. Since everyone is genetically different, some people are better able than others to process sweets. If you are overweight, if any blood relative has had diabetes, and if you suspect you may have hypothyroidism or a sluggish metabolism, you would be well advised to eliminate or significantly reduce your sugar intake.

Too many foods contain sugar as a "hidden" source of calories. Before foods enter your supermarket basket, read the labels. If sugar is listed as one of the first three ingredients, do not put that item in your basket. The ingredients are listed from high to low, according to the quantity contained. Find another product. You do not need the extra calories from sugar. To keep your intake even to a "moderate" level requires constant vigilance. You can find sugar in your food where you may not expect it, for example, in ketchup and peanut butter! If you use an artificial creamer in your coffee, probably most of that "cream" is sugar. Very few breakfast cereals contain no sugar-- some have as much as 50 per cent. Your sweet tooth is an acquired taste. Once you wean yourself from sugar, your taste buds seem to change. What you used to think was just sweet tasting, becomes too sweet-- even disagreeably sweet. I actually can not eat anything with a sugared icing. It is just **too** sweet tasting for me. Fruits taste sweeter to me now and they easily substitute for dessert.

Eliminate refined sugar (and many items with ingredients that end in "ose") from your meals. Instead of eating a slice of bread that contains sugar, eat a slice of bread that contains no sugar. (French bread, sour dough and rye bread usually do not have sugar.) Instead of sipping soup that contains sugar, sip soup that contains no sugar. You will not be changing the quantity of food that you eat-- it's still palm size-- but you will be changing the quality. See if you can reduce the amount of sugar in your recipes by half, or use a ripened banana or substitute fruit juice instead. If you were to get rid of every cardboard box, can, frozen package and bottle in your kitchen that contained sugar what would remain? This is a test of how well you have been eating. Replace these items with products that do not contain sugar. If you take just this one step, I guarantee you will lose some weight simply by eliminating the sugar in your diet.

Welcome water
One of the best things you can do for yourself is to drink water. If ever there was an elixir for losing weight, water is it. Water is good for so many things besides a good

complexion! Basically water flushes the kidneys. When the kidneys are not fully flushed the liver picks up the extra burden. When the liver is asked to do some of the kidney's work, it can not optimally do its job of metabolizing fat. Water will also help to rid some of the waste products from the body that were previously stored in your fat cells. As you lose weight, fat and other substances are released into the bloodstream. You want to get rid of these metabolized products as quickly as possible.

While you are losing weight it is important to keep your bowels functioning normally. Water is essential. If your fluids are out of balance constipation results. With adequate water all systems of the body improve. Best of all for most people, with increased consumption of water, their appetite diminishes. Water is filling.

If you do experience hunger while losing weight, here's a little trick that you can do with water to reduce your hunger and appetite: Add a little grape juice (1/3 cup = 1 Fruit chit) to a glass of water and drink it 30 minutes before sitting down to a meal. Whenever you feel hungry, take this little "magic potion" and the physical hunger will subside.

Anyone who knows me can tell you that I am seldom seen without a cup or glass in my hand. During the summer months I have water with a slice of lemon, or one of the flavored mineral waters with ice. During the winter months I have hot water with lemon or an herb tea. Some teas have a sweet orange spice flavoring that I find substitutes beautifully for a dessert. I am always drinking water, hot or cold. I limit the caffeine containing beverages so that I do not lose more water than I take in. Get into the habit of always having a glass or cup of water readily available. And the old adage, to drink 8 glasses a day in my opinion still holds true. Water has no calories. Drink as much as you like. And like Vegetables it is unlimited. But not to excess either.

For traveling, keep a bottle of water handy. You can take this wherever you go. If you work in an office keep a glass and a pitcher of water on your desk. If you keep your cup, glass or bottle in sight, it will be a natural reminder to drink some water. Drink water before each meal, and after each meal. Instead of snacking while watching television drink a flavored water. It gives you something to do, something to occupy your hands, and something to put in your mouth!

An open hand
The strategy of eating using your hand as a guideline is simple enough. There are indeed some margins for error. You could overestimate how much fits in the palm of your hand. You could make poor food choices. Certainly a brownie as a Carbohydrate is very different from a potato as a Carbohydrate. Milks are different too. There is whole milk, 2% milk and skim milk. I believe that you know there are more calories in a brownie than in a potato, and that there is more fat in whole milk than in skim milk. But I will not advise you to drink skim milk, especially if you don't like it. There is no secret about what foods are considered healthy to eat. To lose weight quickly stay with low fat, no sugar foods. However, even if fattier more caloric foods are included, you will **still** lose weight with MagicHand eating, but more slowly. This is not a deprivation diet. You can choose the foods you want and make the choice-- to lose weight quickly or more slowly-- by the foods you select in each food group. To maintain your weight loss, you can use trading options between food groups, giving yourself even more freedom. Your job is to lose the

weight you don't want and to maintain that weight loss. What makes it possible for you to live with this Plan forever is this built-in flexibility. By monitoring your weight loss, you will discover what liberties you can and can not take. For myself, I know that to maintain my weight loss, I must keep sugars out of my diet. I also know that Fruits are my best friend. When I trade my Fruits for Carbohydrates, I tend to gain weight. You will learn, as I have, how to fine tune this Plan to your own rhythms of eating. You can trade food groups, and you can spread your meals over the day, eating every hour if you'd like. What stays in place is 12 palm portions and 3 thumb portions every day, 3 for each food group. You cannot "save" chits from one day to use for another day. Nor are you required to use all your chits if you don't feel like eating. Every day starts anew with 12 palm portions and 3 thumb joint portions.

Within these rules you have full control over what you eat, when you eat and how often you eat. Give the illusion of being one of the slim people who eats what he or she wants-- the *illusion* of not controlling, of not being on a diet, when in fact you are. Is this Plan too permissive for you or will it enable you to live a life of pleasure-- **in control** of maintaining your ideal weight? I have dared to remove the handcuffs. I trust that you know what's good for yourself.

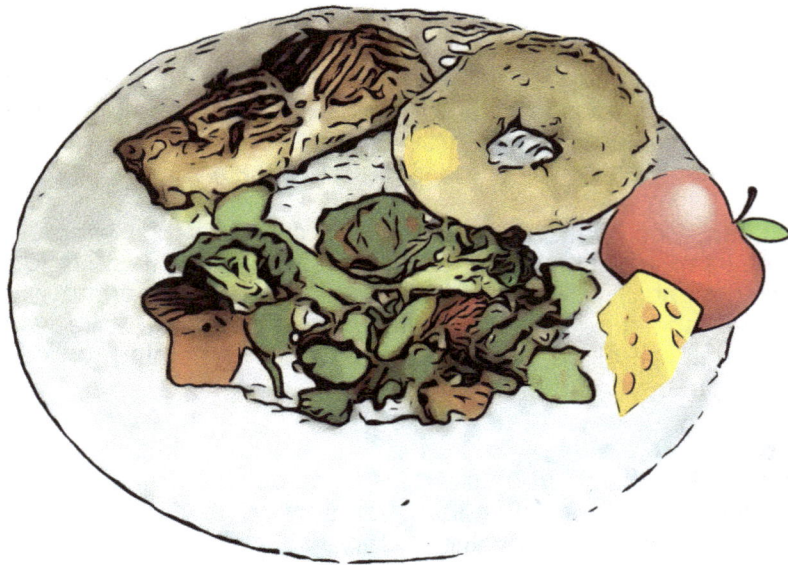

Find the 6 food groups on this plate!

Take away message: After you've had some success, make sure to "hold" that weight loss. It is just as important to maintain your new weight as it was to lose. Do not take too many liberties.

● Point 3: Adapt

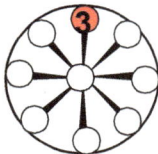

This is a road show

One of the benefits of having an eating plan tied to your hand is that it is something that travels with you wherever you go. Most lose-weight programs do not permit the degree of freedom and flexibility offered here. This program is lifelong therefore it **must** be livable and it must be able to accommodate all the influences, pitfalls, and assaults coming from outside your home. That means no matter where you are-- in a plane, at your mother's house or at a weenie roast-- you can still eat and not gain weight if you follow the principles of the MagicHand.

One of our basic tenets is that you should not feel deprived. In this Point we will discuss how you can have your cake, eat it, and not gain weight. Eating outside your home does not mean that you have no control over your situation. One by one we'll tackle the most common social situations where overeating is sanctioned and even encouraged. You will have to learn how to cope in these situations where so many of the "right" foods may not be available when it is time to eat.

Where most of us have difficulty controlling our intake is over the winter holidays, traveling, and eating at restaurants. Are you ready to learn the tricks of the slim people? Let's begin our journey in the world of eating booby traps.

Fast-food dilemma

Especially if you travel on the road, or have children, fast-food restaurants are hard to ignore. They are convenient, efficient, and inexpensive. More and more fast-food restaurants are starting to offer healthier options and may include a salad bar or broiled chicken. You can balance your meal using palm portions. For example, an order of milk, a small burger and a side salad with dressing will probably cost you four palm portions and a thumb of oil, but you'll be eating from all the food groups, and still staying with the Plan. Hopefully you will feel full enough and satisfied. Fast-foods are to be consumed judiciously, and infrequently, and must be made accountable for the amount of fat, protein, and carbohydrate they contribute to your well-balanced diet. If you can not balance your meal at a fast-food restaurant, and eat more protein or fat than your palm portion would allow, then you can compensate at the next meal by eating very little fat or protein and by eating a large portion of greens.

Traveling on wheels

Maintaining your weight is a heroic challenge for the constant traveler. You are at the mercy of roadside restaurants, train dining or snack cars, and in-flight menus.

When you are on the road, you lack control over your general diet-- therein lies the problem. But, you can put the odds in your favor. Try to keep your meals regular by not skipping any meals. Some foods you can keep supplied in your own car. You'll save money if you keep some tangerines in your car and have one as your breakfast fruit instead of ordering a glass of fruit juice. They keep well and are tasty and filling. Or, you could keep a pack of fruit juices. If you will be traveling for two or more hours in the car, you would be well advised to keep what I call a "snack pack". A quick snack can prevent you from having to stop at a fast-food place because you are hungry. Sometimes traveling another half-hour on the road means the difference between stopping at a greasy-spoon eatery or stopping at a place that might serve a healthier menu.

Your portable snack pack could include canned vegetable or fruit juice, sunflower seeds or nuts, peanut butter on crackers, small boxes of raisins, breadsticks or crackers, tea or coffee and a small bottle of mineral water. All these foods will "keep" for a while and do not require refrigeration. I maintain a pack like this in my car for emergencies, and I regularly replace the older food items. It has saved me many times from having to purchase foods in desperation when I felt hungry. I also know that what I'm eating is healthier than the average road fare. That's a real plus.

In the air

Sometimes airlines give you a choice of several menus and often there is a "lighter" menu and some airlines only offer a bag of peanuts if that! Using your hand to visualize you can keep your portions under control no matter what you select. If you are offered beverages, be smart and order non-dehydrating beverages like mineral water and fruit and vegetable juices or milk. If you order mineral water or a vegetable juice you don't have to give up any chits. And, of course, you could have as much tea or coffee as you'd like, but they tend to be diuretics. Select your foods carefully and count your beverage consumption as part of your meal.

On solid turf

The problem with eating at restaurants is that they generally serve too much food! All the food groups are likely to be represented, offering you the possibility of a balanced meal. To get variety into my diet, I order at restaurants those foods I don't usually prepare at home (or are difficult to prepare tastefully). Rather than to order a full meal, depending on your circumstances, soup and salad and a slice of French bread might be enough. Do not feel compelled to order the complete dinner. If others are ordering the dinner special, you can ask for your salad first and also ask for the soup to be served at the time of the entrees. Ordering a la carte is a way for you to plan your own meal. Just say to the waitperson, " I'll have my soup as the entree." If your companions want to know why you're not having a full dinner, don't say you're watching your weight. Simply say, "Soup and salad are just my favorite thing." Or, "I feel like having a light supper, so I'm going to have the soup and salad."

However, you may also choose to order from the regular dinner menu. You are probably aware that most restaurants still consider meat to be the center of attention, so your protein portion will be larger in most instances than the palm of your hand. Rather than to over-indulge and put on weight that you don't want, follow these simple guidelines:

●1. Immediately, when your entree arrives, take your knife and fork and cut the meat portion in half (assuming it is twice the size of a palm portion). Make believe that one half of it doesn't exist and put it to the side of your plate. You can put that saved half in a doggie bag.

●2. Eat all your vegetables and the salad-- they are "unlimited", but be careful about how much dressing you use. One tablespoon of salad dressing would be one

dr. Anne plan

thumb of salad oil. A pat of butter on your slice of bread would also be a one thumb chit. So, keep counting. If you planned properly during the day, you should have enough chits left (because you saved some) to be able to eat this dinner. At the end of the meal, when the waitperson returns, ask for the doggie-bag and the meat/protein portion that you didn't eat may find itself consumed at tomorrow's lunch or dinner.

●3. Peruse the dessert menu and decide if anything on that menu is appealing enough to use yet another palm portion chit. Some desserts are larger than a palm portion, and even if they fit within the palm of your hand, desserts tend to be rich (over 100 calories) so if you really want something on the menu ask if someone else at the table would be willing to split a dessert with you because you are just too "full" to have a whole one. Most restaurants are very accommodating and will even bring you an extra fork and plate. Do not feel forced to order dessert because everyone else does. You can say, "That cheesecake sounds so good, but I'm so full, I think I'll just have coffee." Say it with a smile.

Keep in mind the example of an ideal meal: Two to four ounces of animal or vegetable protein-- the protein that would fit in the palm of your hand; one slice of bread or a roll, one pat of butter, and any amount of raw or fresh or slightly cooked vegetables and a piece of fruit and perhaps a small glass of milk. That's a lot of food and you do not need to eat everything at one sitting. It's best to eat only as you feel hungry.

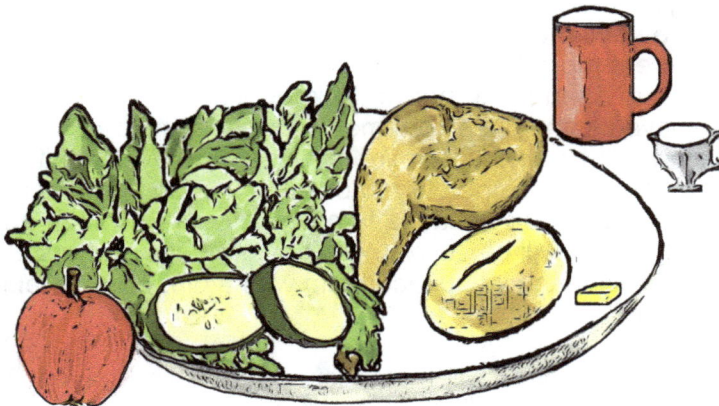

The farther away you get from this balance the unhealthier the meal.

Take your hand with you and plan ahead for eating at restaurants by cutting back some of your chits from other meals on that day. Portion control is the essence of successful restaurant eating. Just because you are at a restaurant doesn't mean that you can throw caution to the wind. Consider it another meal; the main reason for being there is probably to be with other people, not to eat. Eating-out is a challenge that you can

45

overcome. Enjoy the event, enjoy the company, enjoy the surroundings, and enjoy being in control as you place your order. Think of how happy you will be when you've not gained weight.

HANDling the winter holidays

They come but once a year, at the end of the year, starting at Thanksgiving and ending on New Year's Day at which time we resolve to lose all the weight we gained. During the other months of the year, January through October there are also feast days available to us, but nothing as consistent and overbearing as during November and December. The word holiday in itself predicts behavior. It's a day of recreaction, and suspension from normal activities. Often that translates into a day of freedom-- celebrate, honor, and lots to eat. With holidays comes food. And eats are available almost everywhere you go. Offices may have special treats; many organizations and businesses have parties, and relatives send fruit cakes and cookies. It's no wonder that the average American gains from 1 to 5 pounds (or more) over the holidays.

We are in this situation whether we like it or not. So we must do battle to protect our svelte figures. We are armed with our hand! Does this mean we can never eat a meal without counting palm portions? No, it does not. We will talk about special days later. For now let us brave these holidays while keeping our palm portions operative.

Often during the holidays we are invited to cocktail parties and big dinners or big buffets. Everyone is expected to eat and enjoy. To stay on the MagicHand it is necessary to plan your day's eating if you know that you will be going out later to a party. Generally what I do is "save chits". I eat a light breakfast, I eat a light lunch and then with my saved chits (palm portions) I can eat more than I ordinarily would at a party-- but I am still counting palm portions. I bring my hand with me and I know for that evening I can have 8 palm portions because I saved some chits from meals earlier in the day. Usually I try to predict or learn what dessert will be and determine if I need to save a chit for that. I only eat desserts that I like! I do not attempt to try to balance my food groups at a party, but I will eat as many vegetables as I can because I know they are unlimited and they are filling. If you know that a big dinner will be served, don't overindulge on hors d'oeuvres. Eat the carrot sticks, zucchini slices and if you lace them with a dip, count a tablespoon of dip as 1 Oil and fat chit.

Before I go to a party or dinner I will know how many chits I have left for the day so I might leave the house with 2 thumbs of Oils/fat and 6 palm portions. I can remember how many chits I have left for the day, and as I eat I say to myself "There goes one thumb, I have one thumb left. There goes 2 palm portions, I still have 4 left." With planning and practice you will become quite skilled at parceling your portions. Since you probably will have no idea what is in the casserole you're eating or the doctored sweet potatoes or maybe even what the main entree is, do not bother to try to balance the meal. Just eat what you want, but count the palms and thumbs! For example, a palm portion of a casserole dish would be whatever might fit in the cupped palm of your hand. If you are not serving yourself and the hostess places more on your plate than a palm portion, leave it on the plate or eat it all, but count an extra chit. Get it? Count your half glass of wine as a chit.

At the cocktail party count whatever you drink as a chit if it is about a half cup of liquid. Better, however, is to forego the alcohol, and ask for a Virgin Mary (tomato juice with lemon) or a V-8. This way you can save a chit (palm portion) for dinner or an appetizer. You must also learn how to say, "No, thank you." Never ever say that you are on a diet. Once you say that, EVERYONE will want you to eat. I will never understand human nature. From my own observations, people can accept "I am full." "I am saving myself for dessert." "I'm just not a pumpkin pie fan. Thank you." "I'd love to, but I'm allergic to caramel." "Oh, I'm stuffed." "I just can't eat any more." But, say "I'm on a diet." and your host or hostess will not leave until you have a piece! They say things like, "Oh, a little bit won't hurt. It's my favorite chocolate recipe." Then where are you? If you still say no, it's almost like insulting your host or hostess.

Learn the phrases of the slim people. You will discover that many of them are "full" or "will have some later" or "already had some and it was great".

Here are some more slim phrases. During cocktails when appetizers are offered, say "Thank you , but I'm saving myself for dinner." "Thank you, but we're going out for dinner later." Then, at dinner, you can politely decline second helpings by saying, "Thank you, but I'm saving myself for dessert." Then, when the dessert arrives, you can say either "Oh, just a little piece, I'm stuffed.", or "I'd like some, but I'm just too full."
Sometimes food is just placed in front of you. In these situations, you must learn to leave the food on your plate. Count your palm portions, decide how you want to use them and leave the rest! Just say "I'm so full, I can't finish it all." Whatever you do, don't try to explain how you're limiting your foods now because you're trying to lose weight or get healthy-- it's downright boring. Finish your meal with coffee or tea if served, and you can have seconds and thirds of that!

Plan for "after-dinner" parties in the same way. Modify your intake at dinner. Eat "just a little bit" (whatever chits you have saved) and make it last. Keep the food on your plate as long as you can while you talk, taking small bites. Again, we are not concerning ourselves with balancing food groups, just with keeping the number of portions within your daily allotment.

In general, try to avoid the hot fried hors d'oeuvres. Nibble on raw vegetables if possible. And before you sit down to eat keep in mind your palm foods and how you will carefully select the foods to enjoy. It's never a good idea to arrive at the dinner table feeling "starved". Spread your eating throughout the day and snack on vegetables about 30 minutes ahead of the feast to curb your appetite.

The coffee klatch
Part of some business tradition is to bring in donuts for everyone at the office, and at home, for visitors to bring some coffee cake to go with the coffee. Again, you must learn to say no or learn to trade one palm portion from one of your healthy food groups.

If you work in an office bring in a bag carrots, put them in a moist container, and eat one whenever you're hungry. Let them all laugh, and let them eat the cake. You'll be looking beautiful while they make dental appointments. Soon they may follow your lead.

Partying

How can you have cocktails without hors d'oeuvres? Or, go to a cocktail party and not have a cocktail? I think by now you may know the answer to these two questions. For cocktail parties, stay with the vegetable appetizers-- slices of zucchini, carrots, mushrooms and celery-- if available. You really do not want to spoil your appetite for dinner! Instead of the traditional cocktail, substitute a glass of sparkling mineral water with a slice of lime or ask for a Virgin Mary cocktail with a slice of lemon, that's tomato juice (as opposed to a Bloody Mary made with vodka). If there is someone tending bar there is often no problem. If your host is the bartender and asks for an explanation you can say, as I do, "I tend to fall asleep with alcohol." "Or, alcohol makes me sleepy." No one wants a sleepy guest at a party!

Always go to a party with at least five chits. If I bring my hand with me and I know I can have five chits towards food, it's easy to count. As I serve myself I can do so in tablespoons. I know that for me about 2 rounded tablespoons equals 1 palm portion. I can also visualize foods on my plate in tablespoons if I don't want to position my palm over the food. I love going to parties with my MagicHand because it's my secret weapon. People usually tell me how wonderful I look and they see that I'm eating the same food they are. They wonder how I keep so slim. You and I know.

Guesting

Where you really lack control is in someone else's home! What can you do when you are served apple fritters for breakfast? Your best friends may eat this way and think it's just fine. You could marvel at the fritters, and say how wonderful they are, but you're a morning light eater and could you have toast and coffee. Your host or hostess is usually trying to please **you**, so feel free to ask for what you'd like. Survey the kitchen to see if there is any fruit in sight. You can also stack the odds in your favor by bringing a "house present"-- perhaps a basket of fruit and cheese. You can suggest placing it in the kitchen and if they don't open it, say, "Would you mind if I opened the basket and we can see how good these apples are?" Again, don't mention that you're watching your weight. No one needs to know. This is your challenge: To eat well, to maintain your weight, and to use your MagicHand under all circumstances and conditions. Of course, if your hostess serves you a home-made cake, made in your honor, to be polite, you should partake! If you really like the cake, take one piece and eat as much as would fit in the palm of your hand, leave the rest on your plate claiming that your eyes were bigger than your stomach. (Perhaps it could even be saved for you in the refrigerator either to take home or for later.) Count the palm sized serving as 1 Carbohydrate. Or simply trade in a chit from another food group for the larger piece.

If you plan to be at another's home for an extended period of time, you can write a list of your food preferences for the host or hostess to supply. You could ask the host: "Would it be easier for you to shop if I told you what I generally like to eat?" Or, you could offer to go shopping (because you love to explore new supermarkets). Whenever my husband and I visit our relatives we always ask if we can tag along on a food shopping trip. We generally enjoy seeing new places and it also gives us an opportunity to share in some of the expenses. We have fun, and in my opinion, it's one of the best ways to get a sense of the community and see the people who live there.

dr. Anne plan

As a guest, you are privileged to make some special requests, keeping in mind and considering the life-style of your hosts. But, even your best intentions can be foiled. I remember asking for peanut butter, thinking I couldn't go too far wrong with that request. I was wrong. The hostess returned with a sugared jellied peanut butter swirl. The **second** ingredient in the peanut butter was sugar! It was awful. I've lost my sweet tooth, but I did try to eat some of it. As a result I learned my lesson and whenever I stay for an extended period of time in someone else's home, I try to include myself in their food shopping activities or volunteer to do the shopping. Truly, there is no place like your own home kitchen.

In a nutshell
Plan for parties and special events by modifying your intake (saving chits) at other meals during the day. You can not save chits from a previous day or delete chits for the next day. Every day must stand on its own and be governed by your hand! No matter what, twelve palm portions and three thumbs a day, and unlimited vegetables.

Everyone has their own way of modifying their intake. Some people skip breakfast which I don't recommend if it makes you "too hungry". For after-dinner parties I usually forego one milk and my starch and fat at dinner time anticipating the foods that are likely to tempt me at a party. For dinner I'll have my protein portion and an almost full plate of vegetables which I find very satisfying and filling. (I may drink some milk just before I leave for the party if it will take the edge off of any "hunger".) Then I can eat just "a little bit" for appearance's sake. I will eat the carbohydrate that fits in the palm of my hand. This could mean some crackers or puff pastry. You **can** make trades and once you become practiced in the system, your eating can be easily governed.

Inevitably you will encounter people who encourage you to eat even when they know that you are in the process of losing weight. Prepare yourself for dealing with these saboteurs. These people are engaging in a thinly veiled power struggle to break down your resolve. Recognize it for what it is and resolve to win. If this person is your spouse or someone else close to you it may suggest that there are other power issues that need to be addressed as well. You need to put the control and power on your side when it comes to eating. Let them "win" somewhere else if it's that important, but not on **your** plate!

Fast-food restaurants, dinner dates, traveling, partying, and coffee klatches won't throw you off your diet any more. Beware of strange places and use your head as well as your hand. Because this Plan is adaptable, excesses of food, family, and accompanying feelings at social events outside your home can be safely negotiated. It takes practice.

Take away message: You can adapt your MagicHand to special circumstances and occasions in order to maintain your ideal weight. Learn by trial and error.

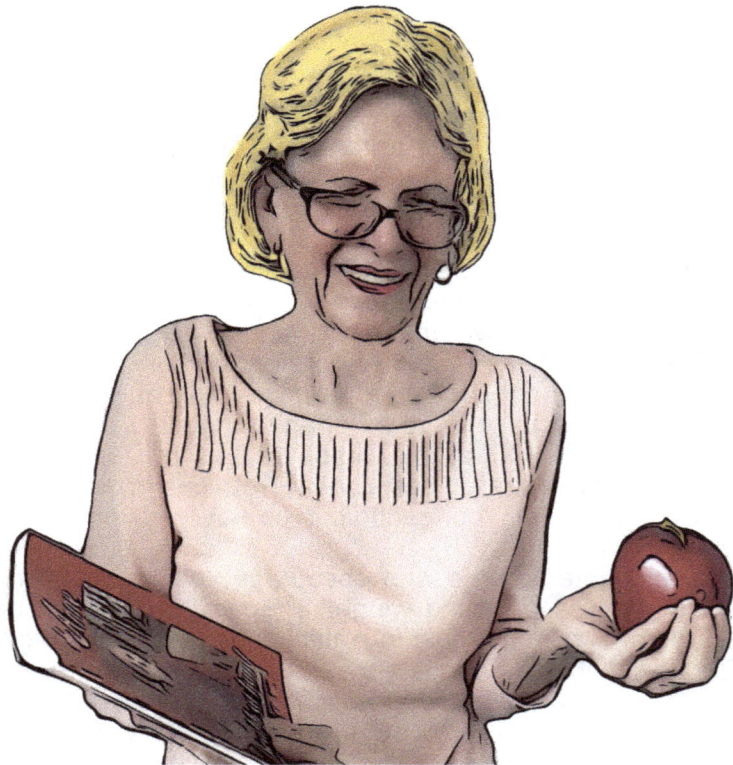

Practice!

MOVE

Point 4: Goals
Point 5: Play
Point 6: Control

● Point 4: Goals

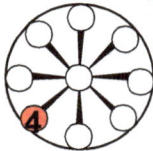

Tuning in to your numbers
To determine what is the best or ideal weight for yourself requires adequate self-knowledge. Very few people have <u>never</u> experienced the joy of being at a desirable weight. It <u>is</u> possible that you may have the so-called "fat gene" which means that you are more likely to accumulate fat than other people. It is well known that **where** fat accumulates on your body is an inherited characteristic. If you have a tendency to accumulate fat, like the alcoholic, you will need to subscribe to a life sentence of watchful eating to stay slim. (Take heart, you have company.)

Unless you were a chubby toddler, and an overweight youngster who never "outgrew" it, you can probably recall when you were really fit, and when you felt and looked good. If you cannot recall such a time, then I ask you to trust that it <u>is possible</u> for you to experience being slim and fit. By using your MagicHand you will reach the "ideal" weight for yourself-- you will have that experience. Natural weight loss that is gradual will bring you to the body weight that is your own best weight, and you will know this because it will be the body weight that you maintain as you continue to practice healthy eating. You

51

will be eating in the general range of about 1200-1500 calories a day which will initiate weight loss, and then sustain the maintenance of your own unique ideal body weight!

For this reason there are two basic approaches one could take to determining ideal weight. It is important to know exactly what that number is because the scale can then validate your eating habits. You can either (1) determine an ideal target weight for yourself or, (2) not worry about a number-- let the MagicHand lead you to a final destination plateau weight. If you <u>know</u> what you want to weigh because that weight is when you looked and felt best, then claim that number as your ideal weight. Eventually-- whether you arrive at this number through the front door or back door-- you will have an ideal weight figure that you can maintain for the rest of your life. Whatever your weight is now, as you read this book, we will call your "starting weight". (Do you know how much you weigh today?)

In addition you should establish an ideal dress size or pants size. You will also be maintaining the same size wardrobe for the rest of your life. Select a "target" outfit from your closet, one that you wish you could wear again and keep that dress or pair of slacks in mind as you lose weight. If you don't have an outfit in that size, buy one and keep it in your closet as an indicator, when worn, of your progress to date. You will see results month after month as the number on your scale declines and your target outfit gets roomier. Then one day you will be there, at your ideal weight. The scale will register the right number and the outfit you selected will fit. This signals the beginning of your lifelong commitment to the Plan.

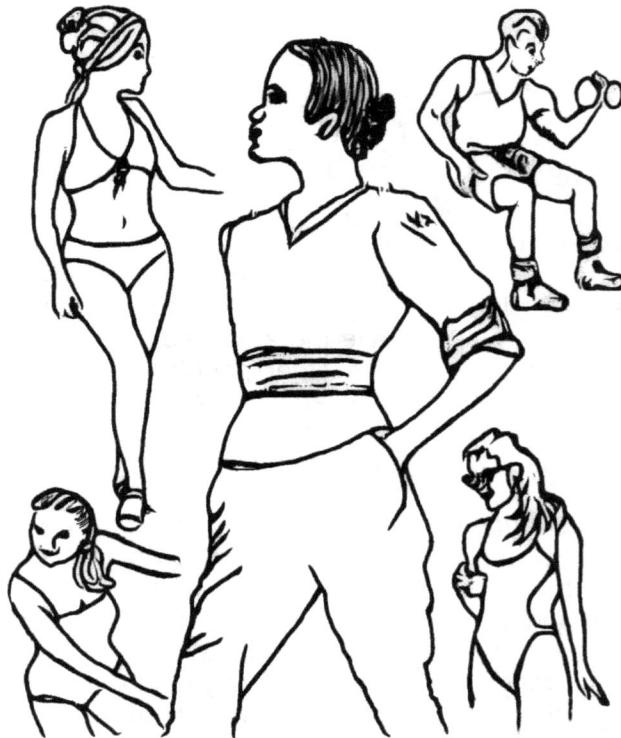

Finding the "right" body for me

Do you have a number in mind? What is your "ideal weight"? Think about it. When you have decided what that weight is, you will establish a range since there are natural fluctuations.

You will add two pounds to that "ideal weight" number and subtract two pounds from that number. So, for example, if your "ideal weight" is 128 pounds, you would have a goal range, of 126-130 pounds. This would be your "ideal weight range". Keep your weight within that range.

Few of us need to worry about going below our ideal weight. Because there are natural fluctuations in weight due to water intake, hormones, and other factors, you need not worry as long as you stay within your ideal range. However, you'll want to stay as close to your exact target as possible. If you get to the top of your ideal weight range it is time to reevaluate your behavior. It's time to ask yourself: Have I strayed from the principles of the Plan? What happened? Did your MagicHand lose some control?

When you find the reason, correct yourself immediately. This is a warning signal that you MUST heed. By the same token any weight loss that brings you below your ideal weight range must be evaluated as well. It may signal some underlying physiological condition requiring medical attention. You are to stay at your ideal healthy weight. If you fall two pounds below, be alerted and if you gain two pounds above, the warning bell should ring. You must be on constant guard and not take your previous weight loss for granted. After you become practiced in using your MagicHand you can become overly confident about your abilities. Because the eating plan is so comfortable and livable you may be deluded into thinking that you no longer need to count your portions. There's a temptation to start taking too many "liberties" with eating because you've been holding your ideal weight. Avoid the temptation to regress back to your old ways-- the lifestyle that helped you to gain the weight. You will discover just how much liberty you can take and it is for this reason that you are given the "warning signal" at a two-pound gain. Remember your ideal weight and your weight range and <u>never</u> allow yourself to get outside that range. This is the commitment you must make to yourself and it is lifelong if you want to enjoy optimal health and slim, trim results. Keep in mind that every body is different. You are the best judge of your desirable weight. (And if you are building muscle you could actually gain weight while your clothes get baggy.)

Accept the truth about yourself. You have suffered from an inability to eat in a way that will allow you to maintain your ideal weight. It is unlikely that you will ever be able to eat without being conscious of your intake because your bodily mechanisms, either physiological or psychological or both, are not functioning towards keeping your ideal body weight. But relax, this is a very livable eating plan. You really will be able to make a lifelong commitment to it without tremendous suffering and deprivation.

Making a pact

To help you make this commitment I strongly urge that you implement the program just as I recommend. Besides determining your ideal weight and mentally visualizing yourself there, I want you to find a "buddy". This is someone who you can trust who will meet with you every month for a check-in. You just need a reliable person who is willing to spend approximately one minute a month with you so that you can verbally tell him or her how much you weigh. This is very important. Your "buddy" is requested only to listen to your report and should not dole out advice or make any comments or suggestions or be critical in any way. This simple reporting requirement will keep you going and force you to be conscious of the fact that you are in control of your weight. Again, this requirement is lifelong. You never stop reporting once a month. Decide who would be a good person for you. Make it convenient for yourself and choose someone who is usually available either by phone or in person. (I "check-in" with my neighbor who I usually see anyway and who similarly gives me his report.) Select a person who is likely to be around for a while, so you do not need to keep replacing people.

I cannot emphasize enough the importance of this little ritual. It will keep you on track. Just think of how proud you'll be when you can report your lower weight each month. And you can be even prouder reporting your weight month after month when it's within your ideal weight range.

Remember it is your weight that you report, not the number of pounds lost. The actual number that reads on your scale is what counts here. To that end, be sure that you have an accurate scale placed in a convenient spot perhaps in your bedroom or bath. Check the reading a few times to see if the type of flooring (carpet or tile) in your home affects the numbers.   You want consistency and accuracy and if you can't get it with your present scale, please buy a new one. Be brave. Step on the scale and record what you get. This is an investment in your future, and you should view your scale as an item that will be with you for the long term.   Get one that works. Because of slight variations in manufacture, it is best to always use the same scale when weighing-in each month. This should always be done on the same day of the month and early in the morning after urination. To repeat, your monthly weight reading should be done on the same scale, on the same day of the month, upon arising after you urinate, and without wearing clothes or shoes-- au natural.

Select a day or date of the month that will be easy for you to remember.   Do not be concerned that there are unequal days in a month or that if you pick the second Sunday of every month as your weigh-in and report date, that the time intervals between recordings will be unequal. Your weight loss most likely will be unequal too and what matters is the trend. You should be gradually losing weight and leveling at your ideal weight. Since this date is a lifetime date, select a day that for whatever reason is easy for you to remember. On this date you will record your weight. It could be the seventeenth of every month or the first Sunday of every month. The only requirement is that it occurs every month and that it is easy for you to remember. You should then report the weight you recorded to your "buddy" as soon as possible.

Assuming that you have identified your ideal weight and calculated your ideal weight range, establish a written record keeping system for each month. How to do this is outlined in Practice Point 4. The value here is that with a quick glance, you can see how you're doing over the months.

You might be wondering why you record your weight only at monthly intervals. While you are losing weight it may take a while for the scale to register the loss. If you weighed yourself every day you would see fluctuations up and down. You may weigh yourself as much as you wish if you can't stand the suspense, but record your weight only once a month. The recorded weight is what counts. Looking back at what you have accomplished is motivating and inspiring. It is also helpful to notice the times when you hit the top of your ideal weight range. Then try to analyze what happened in your life at that time. After a while you will have a collection of monthly entries to document your weight loss and weight maintenance experience. Save them all.

You may start to notice seasonal cycles and even times when you approach the bottom of your ideal range. It's not unusual for people sometimes to go below their ideal weight during the summer months (if they are increasing their exercise activity) and to hit the warning signal at the top after all the December holidays. This record shows your history of weight loss and gain patterns. Well-balanced eating and natural weight-loss is our goal.

Your old actions brought you excess pounds and that's what needs to be changed. What we tend to forget is that people who have problems keeping their weight under control just cannot be given free rein in front of an "all you can eat" buffet. There are people who can eat without overeating. They are slim. They are often aware of when they are hungry and when they are not. Somehow they know when to stop. If we were like these slim people, we would not have this problem! But, we're not, and it is necessary to recognize that fact.

The pill that is so difficult to swallow is that the permanent correction requires commitment for a lifetime because you maybe don't know, never learned, or were not brought up to eat correctly. New habits must replace the old.

Take away Message: Record your weight monthly, make notes— you'll soon learn how to maintain your ideal weight!

dr. Anne plan

● Point 5: Play

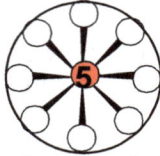

The body good goal

Who wouldn't want a quick simple solution to getting a great body? While you may hear promises that you can achieve great results with one pill or just by overloading on one food, the acquisition of good health and a great body remains omnidimensional. Nevertheless the way to **good** health and **good** muscle tone requires no special apparatus or obscure remedy. But notice I didn't say **excellent.** I'll make one assumption about you and that is that you are not seeking an Olympic gold medal. If you are, then I suggest you stop right here. But if you are not about to compete in some fitness arena, then this is what you must know. With (I'm guessing) considerably less than half the effort that it would take to become an excellent athlete you could become instead a person with a "good" level of fitness. Would you be willing to settle for good over excellent?

For your health and weight control you don't have to overdo it! The goal of **good** fitness can be easily incorporated into your present life pattern and the pursuit enjoyed.

Feeling good

The body works like a perpetual motion machine and seeks habitual patterns. If the machine is set on the "active" knob the body moves in that mode. If the machine is set on the "sedentary" knob the body literally sits in that mode. So, if you sit in an office all day, you are much more likely to continue sitting when you get home-- perhaps in front of a television or computer! To put it bluntly: if you're a slug, your natural tendency is to remain a slug. But, if you're a racehorse, your natural tendency is to keep running.

Changing yourself from a slug into a racehorse requires motivation. But once you make that transformation you will want to stay there. You will look great, feel better and enjoy your new world.

Moderation, however, is still the key. Body damage can occur when we push ourselves too fast, too soon. Ultimately you are the only one who knows what pace is a healthy pace for yourself on the road to physical fitness and the body good goal. Generally regular exercise of some sort every other day or about three times a week is all you will need to keep your muscles and breathing apparatus in good shape. All you really need to do is to add and maintain enough exercise to firm your body and keep it fit. The problem is often not so much what to do but how to integrate regular exercise into your daily living. Physical fitness can be easy to acquire and maintain if the routine suits **you** and makes **you** feel great.

Adding movement

Physical activity benefits every cell in the human body. Muscle cells especially respond to movement. The heart beats faster (pumping more oxygen), the lungs expand (providing more oxygen) and the blood vessels expand (delivering more oxygen) to all the working cells of our body.

With an increase of muscle cells comes an increase of muscle tissue, and an added benefit-- an increased metabolic rate which helps to burn off calories even when you are at rest. The more muscle tissue you have, the more calorie-burning enzymes you will have at work. For these reasons physical activity is an important and necessary part of any total health and weight control program. To repeat, the more muscle and less fat you have, the more energy your body will use--even at rest. This is why men tend to have a higher metabolic rate than women-- they have more muscle to begin with. The longer and more intensely you exercise, the greater the temporary boost in metabolic rate-- basically you are working harder.

Extreme dieting that results in the loss of muscle tissue is therefore counterproductive. What you want to do is lose fat tissue and gain muscle tissue. The best way for the fat person to lose weight is through a slow, but constant weight loss regimen accompanied by moderate physical activity. When you get to the last ten pounds over your ideal weight, then gradually increase the intensity of your physical activity to a level that feels comfortable and that is possible to maintain for the rest of your life.

Physical activity should be used to tone the muscles, not to lose weight. As a matter of fact, muscle tissue weighs more than fat tissue so you could actually get slimmer or firmer and gain weight! (That's why I think it's important to keep a dress or pants size in mind as well as an ideal weight.) If the scale goes up but your clothes look better, then you can safely assume you're gaining muscle tissue and not fat.

The last ten pounds

If you are within the last ten pounds of your ideal weight, congratulations! But this is now when the going gets tough and the tough get going. Literally. It's time to "up" the exercise. Engage in any moderate physical activity that pleases you. My objective is only to make this health program as easy as possible for you. And once you are within ten pounds of your goal weight, your lighter weight will bring relief to all your joints, giving you more energy and the ability to spring your body into shape.

If you are not within the last ten pounds of your goal weight start easy, perhaps by toning and firming muscles. It is essential that you become aware of your body. Correct posture and correct body alignment are basic to success in almost any athletic undertaking. Many people start to run before they can walk straight! Have you ever seen someone huffing and puffing with his or her toes pointed outwards? This is asking for trouble and injury if your body is not aligned properly and one foot does not follow the other!

The pelvic tilt

When we made our evolutionary transition from four legs to two legs, we were left with a weak spot-- the lower back and abdominal muscles. Unless we make a conscious effort to strengthen these muscles, our bellies will bulge and our backs will weaken with any physical stress. Before you engage in **any** physical activity strengthen that pelvic girdle. When you look at yourself sideways in the mirror, do you notice that your abdomen protrudes? If so it could be the result of weakened abdominal muscles as well as some excess flab. Acquiring a strong pelvic girdle will give you almost immediate results-- results that you can see in the mirror.

dr. Anne plan

Now place yourself sideways in front of a good size mirror. Stand straight and see if you can pull in those abdominal muscles and tighten your buttocks. (Get up from that chair NOW.) Squeeze those buttocks as if you were holding a silver dollar between those cheeks. Now lie down on the floor, on your back.

Follow these instructions: Lie on your back keeping your legs slightly parted. To the degree possible keep your shoulders, midsection and hips flat on the floor. Squeeze in your buttocks and press your mid-section to the floor: slightly raise above the floor. Hold to the count of 3 or 5 and release. See the image on the next page.

Relax. Press your spine down. Tighten your butt. Pull in your belly. Lift up.

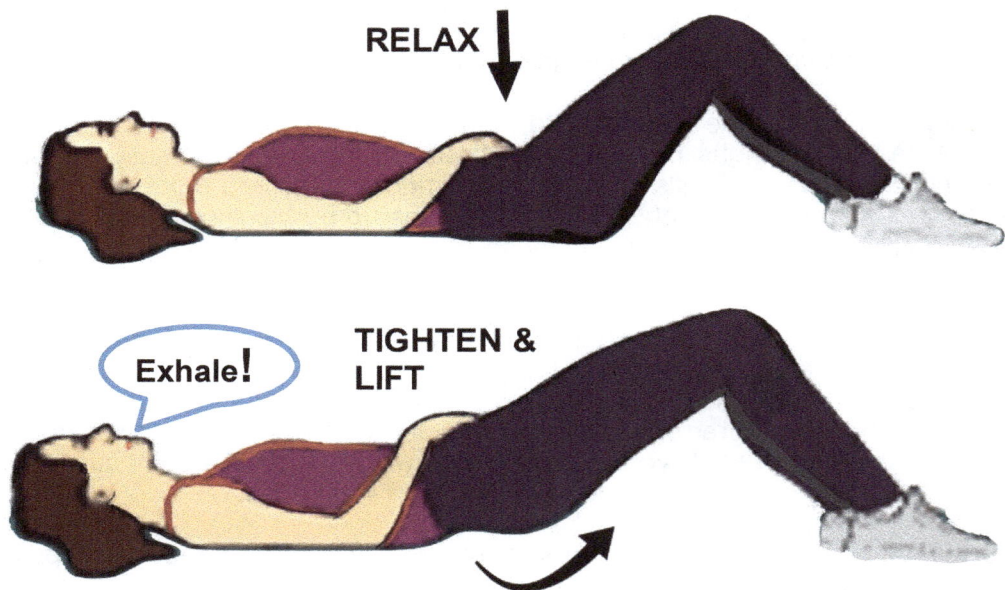

RELAX

Exhale!

TIGHTEN & LIFT

Coordinate your breathing as you tighten and release your pelvic muscles. Always **exhale as you draw in your lower abdomen** and simultaneously tighten the buttock muscles, flattening your lower back. **Inhale when the muscles are relaxed.** In general, whenever engaging in any exercise, always remember that you should be exhaling when the muscles are tightened or contracted and that you inhale during the preceding interval when the muscles are relaxed or extended. Relax and breathe in, tighten the pelvic girdle as you breathe out. This is called abdominal breathing. (If you are inflating your chest and moving your shoulders you are not breathing properly.)

You can practice tightening the pelvic girdle almost anytime, anywhere, any time of day. Perhaps you can lie on the floor while watching television. Whether walking or bending or picking up objects from the floor, remember to keep a tight pelvic girdle, keep your spine straight, and bend your knees. You will reduce your chance of back injury and look slimmer even if you don't lose a pound. Women especially should avoid high-heeled shoes, that is, any shoe with a heel higher than two inches. Check your sleeping position-- a rounded back is best, sleeping on the side with a bend to the knees. Whenever you get the opportunity, tilt that pelvis and tighten those buttocks. Eventually, without thinking, your body will retain the strengthened position. Avoid letting it all hang out!

You can also stand against a wall and get similar benefit by pressing your back against the wall, closing the hollow part of your back. Try this. With the heels of your feet no more than a foot away from the wall, pull in your abdominal muscles and flatten your back against the wall. If you are doing this exercise correctly, your hand will not fit between your back and the wall surface. This is a great exercise to do while waiting for elevators, or, in fact, waiting any place where you can find a flat wall. I often do my pelvic tilt while I am walking or while I am standing in line at the supermarket or at a sales counter. (I use the time!) One woman told me that she does her pelvic tilts while housecleaning. Every time she walks through a doorway, she stops and tilts! As a result, she looks terrific with a firm and flat "stomach". Become conscious of your mid-area and select the situation or routine that suits you.

Some foot-rules
I know that you think you know how to walk. After all, just like breathing, you've been walking just fine. So, let's take the tell-tale test. Find any pair of flat soled shoes (loafers, tennis shoes, or sandals, etc.). Look at the bottom of your shoes. If either edge of the heel is worn down, it means that you are not walking properly. The wear on your shoe should be fairly even from the edge of the inner heel around to the big toe. Stand about five steps away from your full-length mirror again and watch yourself walk. Walk towards the mirror. Do your feet turn outward or are the toes marching straight ahead? Watch yourself. Walk in a heel-toe rhythm with the heel striking first. Your toes should be straight ahead.

Keep your head erect, and arms swinging as they brush against your side. As the left foot advances, the right arm swings forward, and as your right foot advances, the left arm swings forward. And remember to keep that pelvic girdle tight. Walking is perhaps the most natural physical activity for us erect two-legged Homo sapiens. Almost everybody walks and I hope you'll be walking for the rest of your life-- so do it right. Stand straight, keep the body relaxed but erect, throw back your shoulders, pull in your abdomen and buttocks and walk straight. Do **all this** with a smile on your face!

A prerequisite to any strenuous physical activity is mastering the pelvic tilt and a straight walk. Put your body in line before you play.

Stepping high
The main reasons for moving your body are to bring oxygen to the cells through more rapid and deeper breathing, to exercise the muscles beyond normal use, and to gain an awareness of your physical being. When we were children we played in our backyards and in playgrounds, joyfully laughing romping, running and teasing. We had fun! Let us bring back the physical play we once knew in childhood. Exercise need not be a chore. When we exercise simply to lose weight or to satisfy someone else's demands (like a

dr. Anne plan

gym teacher's), what was once fun becomes work. Forget about the benefits of exercise and concentrate on the joy it can bring. Think about it. What did you really enjoy as a youngster? Was it skipping rope? Shooting hoops?

The best exercise for you is the one you'll do consistently and enjoy. I could present a large table describing the benefit of each sport, but I do not believe that any one exercise should be selected over others because of its particular benefit. Physical activity, of almost any kind, will increase your awareness of your body and build your muscle tissue. Do not concern yourself with whether an activity is considered aerobic (without oxygen debt) or anaerobic (with oxygen debt). Obviously, you can sustain an activity for a longer period of time without stopping if you don't run out of oxygen! Many sports combine both qualities.

What's important is that you get out and move. Or stay inside, and move. Truly the best exercise in the one you enjoy doing the most.

And flexibility is important for either aerobic or anaerobic exercises. So, do not choose an activity because it is either aerobic or anaerobic or promotes flexibility. Keep in mind that some people are better suited for one type of exercise than another. For example, if you lack flexibility, you may be more prone to injury if you take up jogging. If you are flexible, yoga or ballet may come easily to you. Some of us are tight-jointed and some of us are loose-jointed. Also, some of us have more sprint fiber than endurance fiber.

But maybe it's been so long that you no longer remember what you used to enjoy doing. It might be helpful to know something about your body type and what sports might come more easily to you than others. Maybe you can tell what abilities you have by identifying the sports that are easy for you.

Explosive ability
Sports demanding this athletic trait are, for example, tennis, squash, football, water-skiing, boxing and racquetball. In many of these sports you may experience an oxygen deficit, making them anaerobic type exercises.

Endurance ability
These sports develop lung capacity. Some sports requiring endurance ability are cross-country skiing, cycling, mountaineering, skating, aerobic dancing and speed roller skating. You will get the aerobic benefit as long as you can still "talk" while moving.

Flexibility
Put your left hand behind your back. Point your fingers toward your shoulder blades. Now, put your right hand over your right shoulder and try to touch your fingers. If your fingers touch or cross, you are flexible. Skiing, figure-skating, wind-surfing, gymnastics, yoga and ballet all require flexibility.

Selecting physical play
Our body type, muscle strength, muscle endurance and flexibility may make the difference in our enjoyment of a selected sport. However, just because it's easier for you to do one thing over another is not a reason in itself to pursue the sport. You might enjoy

selecting a sport that increases your flexibility if you're not flexible or increases your lung capacity if you have low endurance. Just as there is no one magic food that will bring you wellness, there is also no one magic sport that will bring you all encompassing physical fitness.

Your physical play must meet several requirements-- it must be fun, it must be something you can do without too much strain, and in short, it must be play. Your physical play time perhaps could bring back some good childhood memories.

Think back to all the wonderful playtimes you had as a child. When you went outdoors to play, wasn't it fun? Did you play hopscotch, or jump rope, or play hide and seek? When it snowed did you go sledding? And when it rained did you have fun sloshing around in your boots? Or, did you stay inside and dance to music? When summer came, were you anxious to get to the beach? Did you have fun building sand castles and jumping the big waves? What **were** your fun play activities in childhood?

I encourage you to get out there and do what seems like fun. If it makes you laugh while you're trying to do the Charleston, or it makes you laugh when you miss a badminton birdie so much the better for your effort.

Part of the fun of learning a new sport is not being able to do everything perfectly. Keep your sense of humor and compete only with yourself. All that matters is that **you're** having a good time while others are sitting at home watching television.

Identify one sport that you find appealing. With time you may want to explore others. Variety, however, **is** the spice of life and the more sports that you enjoy, the greater will be your choice of activity and the less likely you are to become bored. You can become mediocre in a large number of sports and still enjoy them!

Plan for the season and select some form of physical play that is the most convenient and easy for you to implement in your daily life. Many activities are only enjoyable if the weather is good. I won't tell you to go jogging in the rain unless it is something you genuinely find fun. The season, the weather, the equipment needed and convenience of the activity are all important factors contributing to the desirability of any sport. Convenience and joy are the ingredients necessary to make a regular physical activity program feasible.

Consider your present situation. Do you live in the country or the city? I've discovered that walking out my front door requires very little motivation, and getting into a car and lugging equipment requires more effort and can make the difference between my getting some physical play or not. When I lived in New York City I was able to make use of an indoor swimming pool located between my office and my residence. I would stop en route on the subway, get off for a swim, then I would get back on the subway and continue home. When I lived in San Francisco, swimming was out of the question. The only pools were indoor pools inconveniently located, so I walked instead. But, when I lived in Escondido, I had a swimming pool and tennis courts across the street at a country club where I had membership. When I lived in La Jolla, there was a pool in my building complex. When I lived in Del Mar I bicycled around my neighborhood. And living in Seal Beach I have a pool in my backyard! In New York City swimming was "on my way home" and now in Seal Beach literally outside my door.

Ideally any activity played outside your home or located somewhere between your office and home or within a ten minute walk from your home or office is the one to pick. Convenience does contribute to regularity, but if your favorite activity isn't outside your front door, judge for yourself if the travel time or distance might foil your plans.

Some of the health clubs are so attractive they just might be worth the extra effort it takes to get in the car and go. And some activities are so much fun, these seemingly minor considerations are of little consequence. Know yourself. Select the physical play activity that **is** possible for you to do right **now**-- in this season. If you need equipment or classes or a partner they can be acquired later.

Mind over matter
Perhaps you've heard that famous athletes have used mental imagery to guide their playing on the football field or to better place tennis balls. It's true. It can work for you. Now you can start to focus on seeing yourself with your ideal body participating in the sport you just selected. If you selected dancing, imagine yourself putting on your leotards and dancing shoes, stretching and whirling to the music. Affirm that you will buy or get from your closet the necessary equipment and clothes needed for your selected sport. See yourself as this dancer (or whatever sport you chose) and increase your awareness of others who dance. When you watch television, notice the dancers. See yourself in the role. Look on the internet and browse through the many websites and videos on dancing. Look for dance magazines or through other popular magazines for photos of dancers. Find a hero-- someone you admire who does your sport. Think dance. Visualize yourself following in the footsteps of your heroine or hero. If you were previously sedentary this mental preparation will ease your transition to a physically active being.

You are getting the mental preparation to transform your self-image. You must see yourself as someone who can do this activity, whatever you selected, and see yourself as fit and trim. The action will follow. You can also just go ahead and do it, but it's an easier transition if you can see yourself in the picture first. Get ready mentally, get set with the proper equipment, and you'll be chomping at the bit to get out of the gate!

The right equipment
Committing yourself to any physical activity means acquiring the equipment needed to safely and efficiently participate in the sport. You'll need good walking shoes if you're going to walk. You'll need perhaps a sunhat and goggles, bathing suit, and lessons if you're going to swim. Don't forget good shoes, shorts and shirt and a well-strung racket and balls that bounce if you're going to play tennis. Without the right equipment, you reduce your potential for joy in sport and encourage defeat. Educate yourself on your selected physical play. Even if you think you know how to ride a bike or do yoga handstands or lift weights, read the beginner books. You may pick up a few pointers, but more importantly, the written word will motivate you to act. When I decided to start swimming again, I was shocked to learn that I didn't know **how** to swim. I'd been swimming off and on for years. I took some elementary lessons and discovered how little

I really knew. Techniques had changed and there were new theories on how to place your arms. As a result, I am confident now that I am swimming to the best of my ability although I guarantee there are no Olympic medals in sight. I am a slug in the water! But, I love the sport. However, I did improve my stroke and I now swim by alternating my head from side to side as I breathe which I discovered helped me to relax more. Read about your sport. Get the proper equipment. And take lessons or a refresher course if necessary.

A contingency plan

O.K. So what happens when you're all set to go for that great game of tennis and the heavens open with an unexpected downpour? What happens when a blizzard appears on the slopes or your square dance partner doesn't show up? We can become easily thwarted in our new physical play program by a change in weather or a change in circumstances if we do not have a good **alternative**. It's a back-up, a last resort, a way to maintain your physical fitness if all else fails.

Discover which activities might be suitable for indoors or as a back-up. Again, be prepared. When the weather is bad, use your contingency plan. When you are traveling, use your contingency plan. You can watch televison while riding a stationery bicycle. Or, you may find a video on yoga or aerobic dancing which you can follow at home. There **are** alternatives. You can develop your own indoor exercise program (to music!) by grouping together specific exercises designed to strengthen and tone your physical problem areas. Most people need to strengthen their abdominals, buttocks and the back of the arms to look and feel good. Find the spot exercises that will do that for you and make them part of your contingency plan-- an indoor exercise you can do on a rainy day. Just pick the spot exercises that feel right to you, that are not too challenging, and seem to do some good. If you have a contingency plan, an alternative to your selected sports, neither hail, nor rain, nor sleet, nor snow will keep you from your physical play period.

A continuous performance

Use it or lose it. When it comes to the body that is the message we get. In order to physiologically benefit from physical play, it must be practiced regularly. More important than the specific sport you have chosen or the intensity of the activity, is the regularity with which it is pursued. Fortunately, one need not exercise every day in order to maintain a good level of fitness. Having this leeway makes it possible for us to juggle our schedules. Certainly, you can afford 20 minutes of physical play three times a week. That's all you need. The truth is, you can't afford **not** to exercise.

Adding movement to your life contributes to reversing bodily degeneration and reducing risk factors associated with many chronic diseases. If you **don't** move, the body suffers gradual deterioration-- called hypokinetic disease. Need I say more? Almost all researchers agree that in order to maintain a good level of physical conditioning, one should exercise regularly. However, giving your body a rest between physical play periods allows the body to dissipate accumulated fatigue products associated with increased blood pressure and cardiac output. How often should you exercise? How long?

The guidelines have now relaxed from what they were years ago. Fitness experts used to recommend strenuous physical activity for at least 20 minutes at least three times a week. I think it's still a good idea. But, if you can't accomplish that feat, take heart. More moderate exercise done over the course of the day can also keep you healthy. Walking to work, climbing stairs, cleaning your car, or gardening can meet similar health goals as long as these activities add up to at least 30 minutes a day. For example, you could take a 10 minute walk on your way to work, climb stairs over the course of the day for a total of 10 minutes, and then wash your car vigorously for 10 minutes when you come home. It would be best to structure these activities into your daily routine, so that they will become habitual. Link them to your work break or to something that will generally stay in place. Keep in mind the joy factor. If adding movement during the course of your day simply becomes another chore rethink your activities. Would it be fun to park your car at the end of the lot so that you will automatically walk farther? Would it be fun to walk to a store rather than to drive?

Here is the rule: Every other day exercise for a continuous 30 minutes, or exercise for a cumulative 30 minutes.

This is the minimum requirement. Do what is easiest for you and what you would enjoy the most. It is a matter of planning an exercise routine that fits your lifestyle so that it meets the criterion of either an accumulated 30 minutes over the course of the day or a steady 30 minutes of physical play during the day.

Whatever type of exercise you select or routine you follow, the training effect will not last unless your activity is continued at regular intervals. More frequent, but less intensive bouts of activity are actually better for you than less frequent, more intensive bouts of physical exertion. Take the slow, paced approach, but in order not to lose the training effect, never allow more than two days to pass without some physical activity. Our goal is to establish an enjoyable activity that you can incorporate into your present life at regular intervals.

Body wisdom
The duration of your physical play period will vary according to the type of exercise you have chosen and your physical condition.

To gain physical results, in all sports, the objective is to get more oxygen into your lungs and to move your muscles beyond normal use. It has been said that you must never exercise to get in shape, but that you must be in shape to exercise. You must know yourself and judge whether a physical activity is bringing you, not only pleasure, but results-- more vigorous breathing and muscle power. Even bowling and sailing can be useful activities if you are continuously moving, remembering to breathe deeply and stretching at every opportunity. Obviously, some activities are more rigorous than others. Does your physical activity increase your pulse rate, deepen your breathing and work your muscles? After all, if you walk in slow motion or ride in a golf cart, you'll get no physical benefit. So, when you garden, garden with vigor. And if you decide that washing your car is what you enjoy, do it at a brisk pace-- enough to raise your pulse and work your muscles. Almost any activity can become a conditioning activity if you keep these principles in mind. The more intensive the exercise, however, the less time you will need to obtain a conditioning benefit. You must become tuned to your body and know when enough is enough. Your body is sending messages to you all the time. If you listen you will acquire body sense.

Become conscious of your body's limitations. Never pull or strain a muscle until it hurts. Pain is a sign of fatigue and a signal that you should stop. Gradually build up your muscle strength, only slightly stressing yourself. And always, when you are engaging in aerobic activities, be sure that you are breathing comfortably enough to pass the "talk" test-- meaning that you are able to carry on a conversation while participating in the sport. If you feel exceptionally tired or fatigued after physical play, you probably overdid it. Don't' fall into the trap of over-exertion-- that's how to become a quitter. Remember what you are seeking-- a physical response to a small amount of exercise. I assume that you are not aspiring to become a professional athlete. They work hard and sometimes very strenuously to maintain a competitive edge. Work into your exercise routine gradually and slowly.

Moderation is the key. Learn to recognize the warning signals of over-exertion. If your heart is racing and your breath is short-- stop. Slow down to a comfortable pace, even if it is a slow shuffle. Getting your body into shape is only a matter of training, and you can do it at your own pace.

Use your body wisdom. And don't worry about what others may think. Occasionally I will be outdone during my fast-walk by a jogger or runner or another fast-walker. My natural reaction is, "I'm not doing enough. She (or He)'s much better than I am." Not so. You are doing what is right for you and hopefully the speedy person that passed you isn't straining his or her muscles and is at the right pace for himself. When I swim laps in the pool, the same thing happens. Inevitably someone else will start to do laps with greater vigor than I, and I start to feel inferior, but then I remind myself that my pace is the right pace for me. Don't listen to well-meaning friends, your wife or husband, or athletes. Listen only to your body.

Tapping your toes
You will discover that some of the physical play activities you enjoy are more demanding than others. For cardiovascular conditioning, the four "best exercises" are bicycling, walking, jogging and swimming. Of these, women tend to be well suited for swimming because of their extra layer of fat giving them natural buoyancy. Because of a woman's wider pelvis, she is more prone to injuries in the lower part of the body-- legs, ankles, feet and knees. In general, for both men and women, I recommend avoiding activities with an excess of bouncing or compression severe enough to damage body tissues. Joggers land heel first and the heel withstands a force equal to 150 percent of the body's weight. If you are overweight, this is why you are at high risk for knee and foot injuries. Short men with a flexible and light body type do well as joggers, but tall men may be asking for trouble.

Your energy level, present physical condition and personal idiosyncrasies will determine the physical play activities best suited for yourself at this time. You must learn to recognize what sports are "good" for you. If the activity doesn't feel good or if you don't like it, don't do it. The crucial element is to find pleasure in the activity. Avoid the extremes, become conscious of your body type, gauge your energy level, and your body will stay in tune.

The transition from a sedentary life-style to an active one is often difficult and it is for this reason that we have spent so much time warming up to the idea. I have given you the secrets to success. If you know that you are a person who can dive into a fitness program and stay with it-- more power to you! If, on the other hand, you have already made several attempts at the fitness game and are no longer participating in any physical activity, then I suggest you follow all of these recommendations:

1. Start to strengthen your body in preparation for physical play. Become conscious of your pelvic girdle and strengthen your abdominal and lower back muscles.

2. Maintain your pelvic belt consciousness and practice walking with your body in correct alignment. Check the heels of your shoes and see that your feet do not "toe in" or "toe out". Your feet should point straight ahead.

3. Visualize yourself participating in physical play. Mentally imagine yourself engaging in your favorite activity.

4. Develop a contingency plan for alternate physical play activities if the weather or circumstances change, not permitting you your regular activity.

5. Find times during the day when it is convenient for you to have physical play. If you choose a 30 minute session, I recommend playing about one hour before a meal or 2 hours after a meal.

6. If, once started in physical play, you no longer enjoy the activity after one or two tries, quit! Find another play activity that feels like fun.

7. Be sure to have the proper equipment appropriate for your physical play activity. Read books on your sport for pointers or take lessons from an expert who will not push you too quickly.

8. Start your physical play program slowly. Plan to play once a week at first, and then graduate to twice a week and so on until you reach the physical play guidelines of every other day.

9. Remember this important rule: Every other day exercise for a continuous 30 minutes, or for a cumulative 30 minutes. Establish the **regularity** of your physical play program before you establish the intensity. Because change is stressful introduce each change slowly. Take it one step at a time.

Take away message: Find an exercise that you enjoy and make it your physical play! Commit to at least 30 minutes every other day.

dr. Anne plan
● Point 6: Control

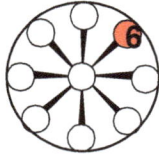

Time on your hands

Funny, isn't it? Who these days has any time on their hands? Most of us are oversubscribed between our work, our families and the various demands of maintaining a household. It would be funny if it wasn't so true. Somewhere in our busy schedules we must find the time to stay healthy. In fact very little time is needed to stay healthy, but to "make the time", a change in routine may be needed.

What is the actual time you will need to stay healthy? For exercise, the absolute minimum would be about 11/2 hours a week in spaced intervals. This could mean 30 minutes of vigorous walking three days a week.

For eating, finding time doesn't seem to be a problem unless you are preparing elaborate menus. Most of us eat regular meals and finding time places no extra burden. Perhaps five extra minutes is needed a day to count your palm and thumb portions. That's all.

For your spiritual health, I recommend 10-20 minutes a day of quiet time, inner reflection, or meditation. How much time do you need to find in your weekly schedule?

To summarize for each week, although flexible, here are my recommendations:

For Exercise: Every other day is about 90-120 minutes/week
For Meal Planning: A guesstimate is 35 minutes/week.
For Meditation: Every day is 140 minutes/week

Total time to add healthy living= Minimal 295 minutes or let's just say 5 hours/week.

To maintain your health almost the greatest allotment of time will go to simply sitting still! This spiritual requirement is what I feel will keep you in balance so that you have the psychological "space" to stay with your MagicHand and the energy and motivation to stay with a regular program of physical play.

At minimum, altogether, you must find about four hours a week to devote to staying healthy. So, the question is, where will you find this time in your busy schedule for the all important task of maintaining your health? Somehow you must **make the time.** The consequence of not taking the time now to integrate health practices into your daily life is that you could spend **more** time **not well.** In the long run you are wiser to allot some time now during the week to maintain your health than to pay later with serious time out from a chronic disease that might have been prevented had you maintained your diet, exercise, and meditative practices.

Any change of routine is difficult because we humans are programmed to be creatures of habit. Just remember that once you get your new lifestyle habits in place, they, too, will become difficult to change. Think about how hard it was to remember to brush your teeth as a child. As an adult, brushing your teeth is almost automatic. If you missed a day for some reason, you would probably feel awful!

What competes with your health time?

For most of us the answer would be either work or family plus internet surfing, video games, clubs, and television. Because our lives are so complex we seem to be in a constant game of "catch-up". I can tell you that I have things on my "To Do" list that are late by 122 days. Lists do help our feeling that we are in control, but they are not the whole answer. We really must discover where our time goes.

For one day, focus on what you actually do with your time. Look for the places where you can cut a few minutes or longer. For example, I have a policy (not airtight) of keeping my phone calls down to ten minutes or less. I also have learned how to scan articles instead of reading every word. My television viewing is very limited, but when I do watch television, my sewing kit is nearby, so I can make repairs. I work very hard to keep organized and to plan my activities in advance. But, most importantly I have made my health a top priority.

An activity record

If you really don't know where your time goes may I suggest a simple exercise? For one week keep track of what you are doing, where you are going, and summarize your activity every hour. Use the Activity Record that follows here as your blueprint. It is divided into 24 lines, for a 24-hour day with enough room on each line to squeeze in four short words to describe your activities. Each column represents a day of the week. You can bracket the hours together when one activity is spread over a period of hours (for example, sleeping.)

My Activity Record

	MON	TUE	WED	THU	FRI	SAT	SUN
6							
7							
8							
9							
10							
11							
12 N							

dr. Anne plan

	MON	TUE	WED	THU	FRI	SAT	SUN
1							
2							
3							
4							
5							
6							
7							
8							
9							
10							
11							
12 M							
1							
2							
3							
4							
5							

Look at all those hours! Where do they go?

Plan ahead
Computers have come to assist us in many ways and one of the best uses of the computer, on a personal level, is that software exists for you to itemize daily tasks and keep a schedule flowing. Decide what hours you have free for scheduling physical play and meditation.

If you have no idea where to put exercise, may I suggest finding a time after noon. Recent research suggests that the body may be an afternoon or evening performer. The perceived effort to exercise later in the day is less than the perceived effort to exercise in the morning. Nevertheless your biorhythms could be different. Select the time that feels right for you.

69

Making lists with or without the assistance of technology helps us to improve our sense of control. And that reduces stress. Finding time in our day can be accomplished, but then you need to find the time to make the plan! Just finding the time to make your new schedule could be challenging. Could you pare down your internet use or television viewing to only those items that are a "must"? Try viewing a television schedule first, then do not turn on the television unless there is something you want to watch. If you turn on the television first there is a tendency to switch channels until you find something that is mildly interesting-- and it just consumes time.

Getting birds to fly
Interruptions while you are trying to accomplish a task are one of the most costly time vaporizers. Two interruptions while you are working on a task can make that job take three times as long. Focusing on your work without interruption is optimal. Take note of how you accomplish tasks and what interruptions occur. You may find it necessary to monitor your voicemails, and then return calls later. Combining like tasks often saves time. You could also ask friends to call you after a certain time if they are interrupting your business hours.

Difficult as this may be, we all must learn how to say "no" to certain requests. Your time is valuable and by setting your own priorities and goals you will know what activities to eliminate. Whenever I feel overwhelmed I think about the President of the United States and wonder how he or she gets the job done. With lots of help for sure. And the President even takes vacations. He/she is highly scheduled. Priorities are set. But In a crisis everything is dropped.

Once you can put your schedule on paper it's off your mind. Develop a possible schedule, one you can live with, and reward yourself by checking off tasks as they are accomplished. The biggest anti-depressant is taking action, and one of the best satisfactions is the completion of a task. You will feel good being organized and actually being able to follow your plan.

Once you are able to manage your time, you will also be able to commit to a healthy lifestyle. Losing weight, maintaining weight loss, exercising, and meditating all require some space in time. You could make no better investment.

Time blocks
To organize your day and to be sure that you include time for healthful activities think in terms of blocks of time.
- First, find where your time actually goes. (Complete that Activity Record)
- Second, can you delegate some activities to someone else who would do it just as well or better? Can your children do their own laundry? Could you service your car at a garage that also washes your car?
- Third, set a block of time aside for no interruptions to get your high priority tasks accomplished.
- Fourth, plan your schedule a week at a time. Allocate some time either at the beginning or end of the week to do this. Make health one of your top priorities on your schedule. Don't sacrifice your health on the altar of work.

- Fifth, follow these basic steps to gain control over your time. Record how you're spending your time now on the activity sheet. Set limits on your activities. For example, if your business meetings take 11/2 hours because people are late, be firm about starting on time and keep the meeting to an hour.

Consolidate similar activities. Don't make five trips in the car if you can make one trip to cover all the bases. File your papers at one time or in a consistent manner. Open your mail perhaps at the same time. Put your paper projects together. Put your computer projects together.

Identify your peak work performance hours. Schedule your important tasks then. Identify your low energy times. Schedule easy tasks at those times, or use that time to regenerate with physical play or stress reducing exercises. Time is all we humans really have. Make it count with days where you get out of bed feeling good and love what you see in the mirror.

Take away message: the benefit of good health is worth finding the time to establish good habits. Make it a priority in your life.

SILENCE

Point 7: Inner
Point 8: Nurture
Point 9: Daily

● Point 7: Inner

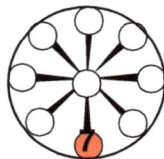

How do I eat every day?

In this Point we will address that part of us that screams to be filled. Or, in other words that part of us that feels empty. It is not enough to know what to do to effect weight loss. You have the facts. You have the knowledge. But there are other factors that need to be addressed to insure your success. Truly the easy part is learning how to eat properly. The difficulty so many of us face is controlling the demons within that may sabotage our best efforts. The need for other's approval is often very strong and the wrong reason for losing weight. Without nurturing the part of us that needs attention, love, and caring, our efforts to lose weight are futile. How we eat, our personal style of consumption, is often related more to psychological factors than the physical hunger we believe we are satisfying.

May I ask, "How do you eat?" On the surface this may seem like an odd question, but the answer may reveal why one is having a problem with being overweight. Whatever you are presently eating and whatever style or pattern you have adopted for meals and snacks represents the weight-gain diet you're already on. It's nonsense to say diets don't work because they do-- either for you or against you. People are frequently telling me that they hate diets and they refuse to go on a diet. What we must realize is that we are already on a diet of our own making. It is "Ellen's put on 10 pounds in three months diet". Or it is "Jack's gain 6 pounds every year program". A diet simply is what you usually eat and drink-- your daily fare. A diet is not a two-week quick fix. We tend to view diets as temporary and negative because they are associated with short-term deprivation. The diet you are already on is what you generally eat, in the quantities you are used to eating. If you are now overweight, your normal diet is probably a weight-gain diet and **that** is what we will modify into a weight loss and maintenance diet.

Some people are lucky and just naturally seem to know when to stop eating and like the foods that help them to maintain good health. These people either learned at an early age how to eat and it's "natural" for them, or by nature were endowed with good genes, a high metabolic rate, and sense. Most of us who are overweight just lack inner controls. We really don't know how to eat properly to maintain our health and ideal body weight. And in many cases our genes are not on our side and our natural physiology is set to accumulate fat. Our forebears survived because, according to biological theory, they were able to ride out periods of starvation during icy blizzards. We who collect fat would be good survivors in the Stone Age. But times have changed. We really don't need to store that much energy anymore and we've become long-lived people. We also know a lot more. We know that living longer and being healthy, feeling good and physically able are all associated with less fat tissue.

Our style of eating has changed too. When we were hunter-gatherers we might have always been a little hungry waiting for the next meal. There were times of feast and famine. In most cities food is available 24 hours a day. We live in a time of constant feast. Only those who are economically deprived face the fear of famine. Ironically, the rich in the United States strive to be thin while the poor often console themselves with food. Our relationship to food in this age many times is socially based.

We have "breakfast meetings", we "do lunch" and we "invite to dinner". Based on physiology and our blood-sugar levels, spacing these meals about 5 or 6 hours apart seems to make good sense. The structure of our eating day tends to follow our natural biology and blood sugar levels.

I have classified the types and styles of unhealthy eating into three major categories: *High Intake Appestat*, *Trigger Food Bingeing*, and *Stuffing Feelings Eating*. (And of course, there is a healthy type of eating, *Healthy Balanced Eating*-- the style of eating that will not lead to weight gain.) If you are overweight, most likely your style of eating is represented by one of the three unhealthy eating type classifications.

High intake appestat

High Intake Appestat eaters are those people who simply do not know when to stop eating. Their physical "appestat" is in the wrong gear. They need to readjust their brains (literally) to give a stop signal at a lower level. These people gain weight because they just eat too much! Or, put another way, they do not know when to stop. They are the easiest to cure, and sometimes they don't need to change their diet at all. Especially for men, regular exercise can go a long way towards curbing extra weight.

dr. Anne plan
Trigger food bingeing
Trigger **F**ood **B**ingeing involves a complicated mix of wrong signals to the brain and psychological dysfunction. People who suffer from bingeing know that they become out of control. The trigger to a binge episode can sometimes be a certain food or a pressure exerted on a psychological button. This eater may eat until feeling even nauseous or sick, but will still want to eat more. If you are a trigger food binger, you know that you just can't stop eating once you start to indulge in some specific food (like a potato chip or one cookie).

Some Trigger Food Bingers are also "Stuffing Feelings Eaters", stuffing their feelings trying fill their "hole in the soul", often not facing their anger. In essence the trigger here is a situation.

Stuffing feelings eating
Not all Stuffing Feelings Eaters are necessarily binge eaters. Stuffing your feelings could be a chronic situation where certain foods are selected to make yourself feel good when what you are actually feeling is too disturbing or painful to acknowledge. A true **S**tuffing **F**eelings **E**ater has episodic bouts of eating for pleasure, perhaps going through an entire pint of ice cream at one sitting when feeling low or the next day eating an entire bag of potato chips to enjoy watching a football game. The Stuffing Feelings Eater is not totally out of control. However, this type of eating is most significantly "problem eating" since ill health consequences may result from being overweight or over-eating. If the physical results of your over-eating mean that you require medical attention (high blood pressure, heart disease), then you are very likely this type of eater.

Learning how to eat will help the binge eater to gain some control over eating. A deprivation diet would be the worst diet for a binger, since as soon as it's over and before it begins two irresistible opportunities for bingeing will have presented themselves. Generally, the binger already feels deprived, so a deprivation diet just exacerbates this dysfunctional type of eating behavior. It is important for the binger to come to terms with his or her feelings if stuffing feelings and/or to recognize that certain foods are physiological triggers.

Psychological counseling is often beneficial. On your own you can document your bingeing episodes, write down your feelings, the time and date of occurrence and the food chosen. You may see a consistent pattern and understand your own behavior better. Ask yourself what you are trying to "fill"? Also ask yourself what you are accomplishing by bingeing. Sabotage? Proving to yourself that you're not good? What? With concentrated self-exploration and the guidance of a professional counselor, you may be able to get at the root of the problem.

Many of us are all three types, High Intake Appestat, Trigger Food Binger, and Stuffing Feelings Eater at different times. Try to determine what type of eating you think is most responsible for your weight gains? Are you simply a Thanksgiving and Christmas overeater who gains maybe five pounds every year? Or can you not be in the same room with a bag of peanuts without devouring them totally and looking for more? Or are you chronically trying to make yourself feel good by overindulging with treats?

74

Mind control

You already know how to eat a well-balanced diet using controlled portions. But you will sabotage yourself over and over again if you do not understand the psychological underpinnings causing your overeating in the first place. So, let's look at all three types of eating to determine what must be done to gain the mind control you need to be successful.

High Intake Appestat:

Your problem basically is that you just eat too much, probably on "special" occasions and in general whenever food is put on the table. Food may be your ""lover" too. You enjoy the company of this food so much that a little more or an extra helping fills a small hole somewhere that says I need love. (Or, I need a friend.)

Many brain chemicals affect hunger and knowing when to stop eating is a message that must get to the brain. Our appetite center is located in the hypothalamus, near the base of brain. Specialized nerve cells monitor glucose levels in the blood signaling our feelings of hunger. Some people take longer than others to turn off the hunger signal or have a delayed reaction to the feeling of being "satiated" and will overeat on a regular basis.

People with a High Intake Appestat will generally have an extra two or three servings at a meal when others around them have stopped at one serving. Are you someone who always has an extra servings when asked because you don't feel filled yet?

Trigger Food Bingeing:

Your problem is that certain foods trigger a physiological response that becomes almost uncontrollable. In other arenas of your life you may also be an obsessive-compulsive personality. In some people, the physiological craving for sugar starts a snowball response to all sweetened foods. Ice cream and chocolate bars are the two foods people most frequently crave. Carbohydrates release the brain chemical serotonin, which is believed to reduce feelings of anxiety and frustration. Serotonin uses tryptophan as its chemical source which is obtained in the diet from poultry, fish, lean meat and peanuts. But these foods must be balanced in the diet with a carbohydrate (like pasta) in order for the serotonin to make it to the brain.

Specific foods, commonly sugar and alcohol, react with chemicals in the brain and can set us up for depression or anxiety after a temporary high. In addition, people may have allergies to such foods as eggs, wheat, soybeans, citrus fruit and milk.

In essence we are all unique chemistry sets. And it is quite possibly true that "one man's meat is another man's poison". L-phenylalanine is the amino acid that converts into two neurotransmitters: norepinephrine and dopamine. The desire for food, not actual hunger, may be a way to appease a temporary negative emotional upheaval. Emotional as well as food triggers are linked to binge eating as with an alcoholic who "can't stop". A conscious and focused effort will be required to control the abuse of (anesthetizing "feel better") food as a solution to psychological disruptions.

Eating becomes addictive because it feels good and physiologically you are triggering endorphins. So when you are feeling down, you may be seeking an upper. The "upper" could be a food that triggers the release of endorphins in the brain, that once started becomes an obsessive demand.

Stuffing Feelings Eating:

Your problem is that you get comfort from food. Food may spell love. So, how can you make yourself feel better without resorting to food? The hardest emotion to shake is anger. And according to psychiatrists repressed anger can result in depression, However, what most people fail to realize is that it is possible to exert control over their moods. I know that when you're so far down it's hard to get up.

The most effective way to lift a depression is to take some **action**--just do something no matter how trivial to solve the problem that is creating your bad mood. (But, don't eat!) If you need some oral "comfort-gratification" make yourself some hot tea or find another low or no-calorie drink that soothes you and drink it through a straw. (How about coffee with a touch of cocoa and some milk or cinnamon to satisfy the "chocolate means love" need?) A long walk might be the best antidote for anger and this makes sense to me. Remember that when we're angry our adrenaline rises demanding physical expression. A walk might be just as good as punching a pillow!

It might be helpful if you can identify your feelings and know if you are angry or depressed. Remember that depression often follows unexpressed anger. So if you **are** depressed, what are you angry about? The chances are good that what we really are stuffing is our anger. Anger usually comes from a threat, a loss, and/or hurt. We can become threatened when someone violates our personal space in some way. For example, if someone continuously stepped on your toes either physically or psychologically, you'd get angry. Loss can occur in many situations. We can think we have failed in some way, we could lose a possession or an ability, or a loved one, and we could lose a part of our life that was important to our identity. Whenever we lose something of value, we might feel depressed. The simple answer is to seek love from a source other than food. May I suggest attending a religious service or listening to a singing group or choir? You might feel "filled" instead with spiritual love. Being in harmony with others whether in a singing group or on a dance floor can fill some empty spaces.

The "need" to eat may be traced to a violation of your physical or emotional boundaries either presently or from the past. You may be eating to add protection-- to build a fence of fat so to speak to protect from further violation. Many overly "sensitive" people are actually people with loose boundaries. Their sense of self may be very open and vulnerable to assault from the outside because their psychological defenses were poorly developed.

Perhaps you can identify some "lost love". Food may be numbing the feeling of the pain of that loss. Food is a lover and eating is a way of coping. Extra fat offers "protection". As one lonely overweight teenager stated, "Look at me. You can see that food is my best friend." Ask yourself, "Am I trying to fill some "emptiness" with food?"

You may see yourself as a victim; you may feel discounted or ignored and powerless. Whatever may have happened to you has much to do with how you have interpreted the situation. The psychological part of problem eating is the inability to express the emotions you are feeling. In therapy the emotional aspect can often be resolved in relation to the event. For someone else a similar event may not have left an open wound. Your healing and the approach you take is a very personal matter.

The chronically angry person usually feels powerless in their present situation, but in fact may have more control than they think. Our feelings of powerlessness often stem from our childhoods even though as adults we are now more in control. Behind most anger is a deep hurt, and if it is intense enough, you may need the assistance of a professional counselor. Dealing with your hurts, healing the wounds, should go a long way towards alleviating the need to stuff yourself with food to avoid the pain of feeling what you don't want to feel. In short, you must learn to stop *feeding* and instead *feel* your feelings.

To summarize, we eat for many reasons. Most emotional eating is fear-based. The threat of hurt or loss causes us to feel anxious so we may eat to "protect" ourselves. After we get hurt, we may become angry and we eat to stuff the feeling. If the anger is unresolved, we may become depressed. If we are lonely because of lost love we may feel sorry for ourselves, and we eat for comfort, or to feel better.

Mood chemistry
Nutrients do appear to impact brain neurotransmitters. As you may recall from biology classes, a neuron is a brain cell. Tiny electrical impulses travel from one neuron to another via brain chemicals and these chemical highways are called neurotransmitters. Your brain chemistry is influenced by what you eat, how you exercise, your interactions with other people and your environment. Your thoughts and feelings are greatly influenced by the chemistry of your brain.

When brain chemicals fluctuate you are likely to experience wide changes in mood. Most women are keenly aware of how their normally sunny disposition can change during a pre-menstrual fluctuation of estrogen and progesterone hormone levels. Although less recognized, men too have similar hormonal mood swings. In general, everyone is subject to thought and mood swings as a result of his or her biochemistry.

Cravings
The brain not only turns your appetite on and off, it also may make you hungrier for specific foods. A blood sample can determine if you have the fat gene responsible for "sugar craving". This gene is also linked to alcohol and drug addiction. In essence the brain is a chemical organ and sugars increase the amount of neurotransmitters giving pleasurable feelings. Your physical and psychological environment will determine to what extent food, alcohol or drugs will be used to stimulate this pleasure center. To abate any substance addiction it is necessary to alleviate the underlying psychological pain and/or find a healthier pleasure substitute. Maybe as the old Beetle song says, all you need is love.

Many people believe that artificially sweetened drinks are the answer to their sweet tooth. Unfortunately, your body knows when it's being tricked, and the artificial sweetener may actually set you up for a real sugar binge. The sweet taste tricks the body into producing insulin in anticipation for calories. When the calories don't appear you may actually feel hungrier. You would be better advised to drink a naturally flavored mineral water with no artificial sweetener.

Jumping through the hoop

So, how can you feel good about yourself? For starters, think about your successes in life. See yourself as a person who is already successful because you are doing the right things for yourself (like reading this book). If there is something that you need to change or improve think of yourself as on your way to that goal. It might be helpful to cut out inspirational or "feel good" articles or sayings and put them in an album or folder to refer to whenever you need a lift. Or perhaps you have a favorite piece of music you could play.

Remember that taking some action will help to counteract bad feelings when they start to take hold. We all face periods of self-doubt, we all wonder about ourselves, and that is human nature and part of our growth process. You must find your own truth to have inner harmony.

Taking control

A growing body of research tells us that personality may play a significant role in health. Emotions and attitude can either fortify or depress the immune system affecting the body's ability to heal itself.

Moods can also be highly contagious. If you are in a "toxic relationship" with another person you may notice that you feel "less than" or anxious or depressed after being with him or her. People who are more empathetic towards others are more likely than others to pick up the moods around them. So, help yourself and others-- put on a happy face!

Self-talk

It is important to address the subconscious needs you may have for actually staying overweight. If you lose a lot of weight and then gain it back it may mean that you have an underlying fear connected with the weight loss. Your pounds may have been protecting you from something. Do you have some inner fear? Who is it that didn't love you enough? The mind will direct the body to gain weight to protect itself. Talk to yourself about your fears. Ask yourself how you can overcome the obstacle, and answer with the solution that you discover from your own self-talk. An answer from someone else may be considered, but put yourself in charge of the final decision. You can solve many of your own problems through this simple process of self-talk, in which I believe most children freely engage, but adults tend to neglect.

Everyone has ups and downs in life. Think of what you can say to yourself to bring yourself "up".

The magic key

The way you behave, the way you think, and the way you feel directly influences your physical being. Ultimately **you** must make the decision to change your injurious behavioral habits and adopt new behaviors for a healthier eating lifestyle. I can give you all sorts of suggestions, and provide a blueprint, but nothing will happen until you decide to take hold of your life. You have the power to change yourself. You simply must decide to make it happen. Ask yourself over and over again how you can make this basic lifestyle program your way of life, how you could make it fun for yourself, and how you could not feel deprived. When you get the solution to an obstacle, then test your answer.

Let me tell you how a little self-searching can work in a positive way. I had a terrible problem keeping track of what seemed like an unending stream of papers entering my office. (My office is in my home.) The problem was that I hated sorting through papers and it was difficult for me to take action on so many things I received in the mail. I kept putting off responses to business correspondence and social invitations and I felt bogged down. Plus, occasionally I'd lose a check! Finally one day **I decided** that I had to find a solution to this problem. Nothing I tried had worked. But I had never tried to make sorting papers fun. What could I do to make this horrible (for me) task fun? I tried to think of what would be fun. I like to dance. Was there some way I could combine the two? My answer was to set a timer for one hour and see how many papers I could clear up in that time. As I sorted papers, I would dance in-between tasks to music playing softly in the background. It felt wonderful to get things done! I now love what I call my "paper hour".

You must decide to conquer whatever could be holding you back from successful weight loss and find your own happy solutions to psychological, attitudinal or relationship obstacles. Keep asking yourself questions (What am I feeling? Can I find comfort when needed by doing something other than eating?) and you will discover the answers. Take a walk. Smell the roses. Take a bath. Talk to a friend. Be determined.

Make the **decision** to go for victory. Don't stuff. Take action.

Take Away Message:
Get in touch with your feelings and see if they influence your eating.
Acknowledge those feelings and find another way to release them.

• Point 8: Nurture

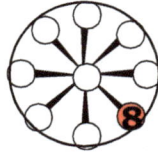

The magic power of meditation

Stress, physical or psychological, can wear you down. Simply defined stress is any condition that impinges upon the organism, requiring an adjustive reaction. Selye, the father of early stress research, defines stress as "the non-specific response of the body to any demand placed upon it ". It is any change--positive or negative-- that requires adjustment or adaptation.

Nurturing is the antidote to stress. It is any supportive environment that contributes to survival-- ones ability to adjust and adapt. Quiet time or meditation provides the stage for decompression, for a natural restoration of calm. Physical exercise is also an antidote to stress. At the right level, exercise produces a degree of protection against stress. Neuromuscular tension can be relieved through physical activity. On the other hand, physical over-exertion, just like emotional stress, can exhaust the body, making one again susceptible to illness. The key is to exercise intelligently--moderately-- so that the body remains in the stage of resistance, built up to cope with stress and ward off disease.

The symptoms of too much stress (over-exertion and tension) cause the distress of depression, fatigue, backache, loss of sleep, losing or gaining weight, irritability, headaches and a variety of immune system-related illnesses. Stress from physical exertion due to too much exercise can result, in some cases, in total physical collapse.

The most common stress, however, is the emotional tension that at day's end leaves us tired. If you feel drained much of the time, get colds whenever they are going around, and lack the motivation to stay with a health program, you may need an antidote to either physical or emotional stress.

Challenge

Environmental challenges to our bodies and psyches can be beneficial or harmful. Some physical and mental stress is necessary to keep us well. Too little stress, called "underload" creates boredom and frustration resulting in the same ailments as "overload". People enjoy challenges and generally are motivated to achieve, accomplish, and to succeed. Too much striving, however, can throw us off balance and our bodies scream "Halt!" If we pay no heed we're likely to get sick. That's one way our body enforces "Stop."

The endocrine system of ductless glands (which includes the pituitary, adrenals, thyroid, parathyroid, sex glands, and the pancreas) interacts with the nervous system to bring about homeostatic responses of the body. Stressful situations tax both the nervous and endocrine systems-- essentially the two systems that coordinate the physiological functions of the human organism. And if the stressor persists, the organism may be forced beyond the limits of its ability to adapt. At any rate, there is no doubt that high levels of emotional tension increase one's susceptibility to illness.

Stress if not managed can lead to ulcers, heart attacks, and other diseases. Stress, if managed, can keep you alive and vigorous, enjoying the pleasures and challenges of life. So, how can we cope with the stressors in our lives?

Concerns about our love-life, work situation and money probably account for most, if not all, the emotional stress in our everyday living. Many live in fear of failing in all three. Others know how to find peace. At home do you find love? At work do you find satisfaction? And in your checking account do you find enough money to pay your bills? Examine these three arenas and observe when you feel frustrated, angry or depressed.

Heartstrings

It's true. Happy lovers do live longer. Unresolved, uncertain and difficult love relationships can harm your health. In a study of stress-related illnesses, various life change events were analyzed for their impact on health. The three events at the top of the list-- showing the greatest impact on health-- were death of a spouse, divorce, and marital separation. Change, whether it is good or bad for you, is stressful to the biological organism and stress can make you more susceptible to the onslaught of disease. Loss of a loved one is especially traumatic. We fear disappointment in love and are reluctant to take the risk of entering into love relationships-- we have the "fear of losing". Though there is no greater stress than the disruption of an established relationship, there is also no greater reward (or calm) than the continuation of a mutually satisfying relationship. Love is a double-edged sword. With love, you can combat stress and conquer fear.

Good friends, like caring lovers, are invaluable resources in life. Married people and people with good friends, sharing a sense of community, live longer than those who are uncoupled or friendless. For the many centenarians living in the Republic of Georgia, a person's wealth is determined by the number of human relationships she or he can establish and maintain. With love and with friendship you can light up your life.

The physical side of love also keeps us healthy. From touching and hugging to sexual intercourse, there are real body benefits: deeper breathing, increased stimulation and circulation. Even a tender embrace can have an astonishing therapeutic effect. Touching is so important to our well-being that infants deprived of tactile stimulation, although well nourished, can become sickly and die. Hugging is an antidote for stress. Allow your mind and body to relax in the luxury of love.

Breathe in love and exhale stress.

Working well

Stressful jobs tend to be those with long working hours that are either fast paced or filled with repetitive boring tasks. Many service-oriented jobs are high-stress jobs. Secretaries and nurses, because much is demanded of them and they have very little control over their environment, lead the list of individuals in stressful jobs. If you can manage your job stress, it will keep you alive and vigorous. You will have turned a burden into a benefit and your job will be a pleasure and a challenge, a source of healthful stimulation.

We must learn to listen to our inner stirrings. A job that nurtures you is fulfilling and rewarding. You have more energy at the end of the day than you had at the beginning. A job that depletes you is one that takes away your energy and leaves you empty. (And food may be filling that spot.)

One of my first jobs after I finished graduate school was a middle management position for a county health service. I was constantly frustrated because I felt the tremendous responsibility of the job but did not have the authority to implement solutions to problems. It was at this time in my life that I had to take the most sick leave from work. I also experienced vision problems, developed dental problems, and gained weight rapidly. (Subconsciously, my added weight gave me the "authority" I needed!)

A frustrating job fraught with tension will wreak havoc with your well-being. You may find it necessary to change jobs or to restructure your present job to maintain your health and sanity. I know such things are easier said than done, but your future health, your well-being, your happiness and your longevity depend upon your actions today.

Tell your boss when a demand is unreasonable. Set realistic deadlines for yourself. Structure your job so you can get the satisfaction that success brings. Also take time during the workday to relax. In between phone calls, roll your head and neck in a circle almost touching your shoulders. And spend a few moments enjoying the release of tension.

During your lunch break (or coffee break) rest your eyes. Sit quietly, close your eyes, and simply cover them with the palms of your hands. Your hands are stress-reducing tools too! This exercise, called "palming", should be done in a comfortable position-- with your elbows supported and with your neck in line with your backbone. Loosely cup your palms over your eyes and enjoy this sweet warm rest. In about ten minutes, having stimulated the circulation by relaxing your eyes, you will be ready to return your eyes to your computer screen.

Another excellent antidote to stress is oxygen. When you feel overwhelmed by the stress and tension of your work and you need quick relief, reach for oxygen. Stop whatever you are doing, collect yourself, and take three long, slow, deep breaths. And when you are about to face a potentially stressful situation, these long, deep breaths can prevent tension build up. The next time you face an upset manager (or your child has dumped a sack of flour on the kitchen floor) pause before you act; breathe deeply and allow the oxygen to bring you calm. It takes only a few seconds and it works.

To the bank
When you don't have money to take to the bank, money becomes an overriding concern. Our feelings of security and control can be undermined by a lack of money. Don't allow life to take you. Stay in control; be the master. If you are pressured by money problems you are either spending more than you have or want more than you can afford. Live within your means and if necessary learn to do without. Place a restriction on any new purchases, sell any extraneous possessions you can bear to part with, and one by one pay the outstanding bills until you can relax once again.

Take charge of financial matters by writing down and itemizing your outstanding debts, plans for payment, and expected future income. This simple act will reduce your financial problems to a sheet of paper. They may not go away immediately, but the facts and figures will be there for you to analyze. By looking at the facts on paper, you de-emotionalize them-- what seemed overwhelming in your imagination becomes something you can analyze and hope to control. The very process of writing down a problem and listing potential solutions can reduce stress. This process is especially helpful if you find yourself unable to sleep at night. The proper place for a problem is on a sheet of paper. You can quite literally put it away before you go to bed and get it out again for further consideration at an appropriate time later.

It is virtually impossible to eliminate all stress from your life, but you can learn to manage stress. Feeling **in control** is key. Of course, we are all different. What is stressful for one person, may be a healthy challenge for another.

Clearing the mind

The prolonged stresses associated with daily living can sap us of our energy. Here are some ways to keep an even keel and take the wind out of the sails of stress. We can (1) change our perspective on life, (2) structure our days to gain control, (3) build up our resistance to fatigue by maintaining good health, and (4) nourish our psyches through meditation. Let's take a better look at these:

(1) Develop a perspective on life that allows you to focus on life's rewards and take its pains in stride. Learn to choose which stresses you will react to and to differentiate between large and small ones. A late appointment is a small stress while the loss of a family friend or favorite pet is significant. These situations do not deserve the same emotional intensity-- don't give it to them.

You can overcome the small stresses by acknowledging that they are exactly that-- small stresses. What's the point of getting angry if your date is a half hour late for lunch? Anger won't shorten the wait. It will only raise your blood pressure, making you the victim. If you're left waiting for a half hour, you can choose to get upset or to pass it off lightly. And don't worry about the "wasted time"-- you can do some pelvic tilt exercises while you're waiting! So, sigh a deep sigh, breathe in that oxygen and put a smile on your face. Then decide when late is "too late" and relieve yourself of the obligation of waiting any longer. Laugh at your predicament, eat your lunch, and take advantage of this opportunity to be alone with your thoughts. Maintain a sense of humor and don't give events more importance than they deserve. Should your lunch date appear when you're half way through your meal, feel free to leave when you're finished. Take care of yourself. Your time is valuable. And be aware that others may not be considerate-- a reflection on them not you.

Another small stress that often becomes major is fighting traffic. My teeth used to clench, my heart pound, and my blood pressure rise every time I was caught in a traffic jam. Then one day I realized that instead of being annoyed, I could use the delay to collect my thoughts or tune in a favorite radio station. I realized I had control over my own reactions. Now, when I'm in that stop and go traffic, I breathe deeply, look around me, and smile. I know it's one of those small stresses that doesn't deserve a lot of my energy, so I might as well sit back, relax and enjoy the extra travel time. Simply some things are out of your control. Recognize when they are. Allow extra time if you can when traveling on the road. It usually pays.

Save your angst for the major stresses that come to us simply in the course of living and loving. The loss of a loved one is difficult for most of us to handle. In this situation acknowledge that you are facing a highly stressful, major life change. Allow yourself the full range of emotions-- go ahead and cry, feel sad, experience your grief. Putting up "a good front" will only add to the tension. During this healing time, you may find spiritual communication, the love of others and quiet times by yourself most beneficial. Keep your life at status quo-- "on hold"-- until you recover from the trauma. Resist the temptation to follow the advice of well-meaning friends who suggest yet other major life changes as a cure. Pull in your horns and come out when you're ready.

(2) Many small stresses can be structured away. We gain control over our lives by organizing our time, planning a schedule and writing things down-- be it in a calendar book, a list of "things to do" or a five-year business plan. Assign priorities to your activities and don't overcrowd the agenda. Structure your days and see to it that every day includes some "free time". If you get fun out of reading poetry (or drawing cartoons, or reading mail order catalogues, or arranging flowers), do that during your free time. Do something for joy. Every day should have some fun time along with those stressful uncontrollable moments we all face. Structure your days, weeks and months to give yourself those fun times-- after all you are the one in charge of your own time.

(3) Of course, the best defense against being worn down by stress is a good offense. Good health and physical fitness give you staying power to cope with life's challenges. Prolonged stress can lead to exhaustion, resulting in sickness, but a healthy body has reserves.

When you feel your body tensing, shake it out. Wiggle your arms, legs and head. Any physical activity will be helpful. And lack of physical activity can be detrimental. The next time you are tense, go for a walk and see how much better you feel.

Discover what soothes you. Our rewards are those activities which nourish the self. We can relieve stress by physically indulging ourselves (I don't mean eating!): bathing in a hot tub, sitting by the fire, relaxing in the sun or in a sauna, napping while wrapped in warm towels, getting massaged, or listening to music-- a rhythmic soothing melody.

(4) The healing silence of meditation can restore your health and vitality. The physiological benefits of meditation have been well documented.

Meditation is a simple way to relax, a way to find quiet time-- there's nothing mysterious about it. In meditation, your goal is to reach an alpha state brain rhythm and to clear your mind of all thought. The purpose is to achieve a peaceful inner calm and balance in your life. Techniques of meditation are offered here for your experimentation.
Find the one that appeals to you the most or develop your own.

One common form of meditation is to devote your attention solely to breathing. In a lotus position, legs crossed and back erect with palms open, the focus is on the two tones of breathing-- in and out. Some meditate using a mantra, which is a word or sound repeated over and over again. Popular word sounds are those with "m" sounds, like "om" believed by some to be a healing vibration. Reciting this mantra sweeps away other thought. The purpose of focusing attention on either breathing or a mantra is to achieve inward centering. Oddly enough, watching television can also produce an alpha state and bring relaxation, that is, if you don't involve yourself with the program but simply allow the sounds and motions to occupy your mind, excluding other thought.

The meditation I recommend is particularly well suited to practicing before you go to sleep. It allows you to dissolve depression, aggravation and tension by sending your troubles away.

Triple phase power meditation
Get yourself into a comfortable position with your back straight either sitting in a chair or lying on the floor with knees bent, feet on the floor. Close your eyes and breathe slowly and deeply. You are now ready to experience the three phases in this meditative process: disposing of the past, becoming aware of the present, and relaxing the muscles of your body.

Phase 1.
        The purpose of the first phase is to bring yourself to the present by disposing of the past. While you are relaxed with eyes closed and hands clasped across your midsection focus on the events of the day. Watch yourself arise in the morning, eat breakfast, get dressed, etc.-- follow your actions throughout the day. View the events of the day as if you are watching a silent movie. Do not dwell on problematic parts of the day or delve into meanings. Think only in terms of events. For example, if you have an argument don't relive the emotional warfare. Say to yourself "And then I saw Sally and we had an argument and then I left the supermarket with the groceries for supper tonight", etc. Observe yourself with emotional detachment. If you find an event particularly disturbing, label it as a "bad scene" or "a disruptive mess". Go on and bring yourself right up to your present place by reciting the most recent events. For example: "I hung up my clothes, brushed my teeth and now I am here lying in bed." Take the day, wrap it in a package, tie it with a knot or bow and throw it away. The day is over and you are here now. You have cleared the day. Tomorrow will be a new day.

Phase 2.
        Place your arms alongside your body, hands relaxed, palms up. This time is for "nothing". The day is gone. What remains is the now: peace and calm. With your palms facing the sky, it can also be an inspirational or spiritual time. It is a time to receive, to be here. Lie quietly, with no thoughts, until you feel "full". Tune in to the rhythm of your breathing. Enjoy the pleasure of being.

Phase 3.
        Bring your hands back to a clasped position over your stomach. Go over your entire body from head to toe and see if you might identify some tense places. Then, RELAX. Go through your body again from toes to head. Any muscle that you find that

feels tense, RELAX. Breathe. Visualize your body as relaxed and at your ideal weight. Affirm to yourself: "I am ...... pounds (insert the number)". Go through your body and see your ideally well-defined form.

This meditation is one I developed to combine clearing the mind, relaxing the body, and using affirmations. It is a "hybrid" combining several different approaches. Feel free to add or alter the components as you wish. It must serve you. Practice your meditation at any time of the day. If you are a person who has difficulty getting to sleep, meditation is particularly good to practice before going to bed.

This Triple-Phase-Power meditation should be practiced every day for at least 15 to 20 minutes. It will help you to more easily adapt to the many lifestyle changes we are introducing-- changes in eating habits and changes in exercise.

We know that any change in your life pattern-- whether it brings pain or pleasure, benefit or harm-- is likely to bring stress as well. And we also know that habits are nature's way of incorporating efficient behaviors into that pattern. When you do something automatically, having made it a habit, you conserve energy, save time and avoid stress.

Transforming new behaviors into habits is a gradual process, and it usually works best if only one or two new behaviors are introduced at a time. It's estimated to take a consistent 21 days of practicing any new behavior to form a habit. Organize and simplify your life, making room for your psyche to absorb changes-- gradually with a minimum of stress.

Again, try to simplify your life and incorporate changes one at a time. For example, when you are about to have visitors from out-of-town, don't decide to hire an interior decorator to go over a new plan for the living room. The impact of your visitors on you lifestyle is enough stress for the week. Find the calm periods in your life to introduce change.

The peace of meditation will give you the support you need to accomplish the changes in lifestyle that you desire, comfortably, easily.

Look at the glass as half full. And take a big drink.

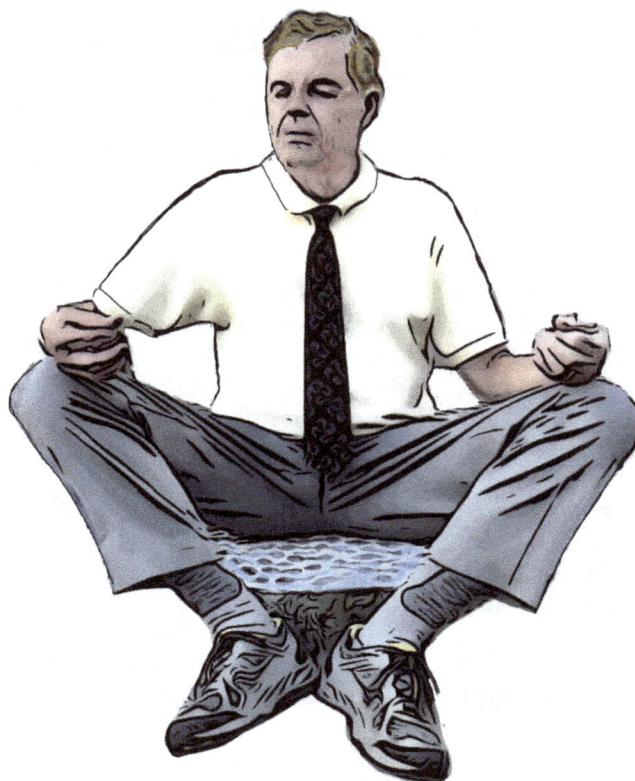

Take away message:
Slow breathing and relaxation contribute to good health. Find the time to meditate and nurture your soul.

dr. Anne plan

● Point 9: Daily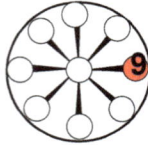

The long view

You say you want to stay slim and be healthy for the rest of your life. If so, what are you willing to do to achieve that goal? What I have discovered is that most people **say** they want to lose weight, but may hesitate when it comes to committing to a lifetime of monitoring. The ex-alcoholic knows that he or she has to practice avoidance of alcohol for the rest of his life. People with life-threatening disorders often have to accept a lifetime of saying no to certain foods or activities. The diabetic knows that he or she cannot eat large quantities of sugar.

What do you know about yourself? You know that left alone like a free range chicken, you are likely to gain weight eventually reaching an unhealthy proportion. Here I assume you are reading this book because you **do** have a weight problem. The last thing many obese people want to do is to change their eating habits forever. They are happy to take a pill, slurp down diet shakes, and do almost anything, including stapling their stomachs, to avoid the necessity of changing the way they eat real food!

We all know probably at least one person who has tried and tried again to lose weight to no avail. The truth is that some people want to keep their problem! To lose weight permanently you must be willing to give up the weight you are carrying and you must be willing to change your eating habits for a lifetime.

For healthy and permanent weight loss results, get off the yo-yo weight loss-weight gain seesaw, and vow to change your eating habits. You will feel so much better. Don't resist, commit.

Pushing on a rope

A friend asked me how I "make" people lose weight. He told me about a fellow who tried every diet imaginable, but who still couldn't lose weight. So, he wanted to know what do I do that's different, how can I make someone lose weight. Unless the person **decides** that it is in their best interest to lose weight no diet in the world will yield permanent results. You must decide for yourself that you want to lose weight first. Then you must select the program or diet that suits you. The quick fixes, two-week restriction menus, are unlikely to work for the long term.

What makes this program your ticket to success is that it is geared for a lifetime, it is easy to use, and most importantly it is extremely flexible. Unlike others, your MagicHand can adapt to almost any situation. Even if you found yourself locked in a room with a carton of chocolate bars for a day, you could still use your MagicHand; count 15 thumb size chits and you're done. That is why you will find success with this Plan. (Remember concentrated sweets fall under the Oils & fat category ruled by your thumb portion). Wherever you go you will always have the tool you need, your hand, with you. Once the program is internalized and you have learned the food groups and how to gauge portion sizes, you will be relying on your **knowledge** of how to eat, and not on any tables or scales for weighing foods.

What will motivate you to commit to this Plan? From my observation the two most powerful motivators to lose weight seem to be (1) the experience of having had a heart attack or (2) the anticipation of getting married. Health and vanity-- both are motivating. They are good reasons to lose weight. What's yours? Right now answer this question. Why do you want to lose weight? Will it take a heart attack to move you or are you ready to make the commitment now?

The answer must come from within. The decision to commit to this program must be for the rest of your life, every day. The rewards of following this Plan will bring you improved health and happiness. I remember what it was like to go shopping for clothes and each time having to try the next larger size. I hated looking at myself in the mirror and it was downright depressing and humiliating not to be able to zip a zipper. Slacks never looked good. I longed for the day I could wear a blouse tucked into the waistband. Now when I look at my clothes I know that I have earned the right to wear them. My clothing size has remained the same since reaching my goal weight in the 1980's. If for no other reason, I am economically motivated to stay slim. The clothes I have I love, and I want to keep wearing them and looking good. I have committed to stay this wonderful size, and that's one reason why I stay on my own Plan. I practice what I preach. Yes, I enjoy looking good. I also enjoy feeling healthy. I have noticed that whenever the calorie-dense foods start to creep into my diet (especially over the December holidays) I truly do not feel as well. It is motivating for me to feel light, to feel healthy, to feel alive, and the closer I follow the MagicHand the better is my feeling of well being.

But to get to these rewards, you must decide to eat according to the principles of the Plan. If you don't do it, you won't get the reward. Simply put: If you eat all you want, you won't look the way you want. If you want to look the way you want, you can't eat all you want. You would not be reading this book if you were able to control your weight at a desirable level without monitoring your intake. Yes, you **could** exercise more, and that will help, but it probably will still not be enough. Decide right here and now that you are a person who will commit to keeping your weight under control by monitoring portion sizes. I have told you how, I have pushed on the rope, but for you to move forward, you must take up the slack on the other end.

It's on the record

Remember the weight record we discussed that's in Practice Point 4? This history is also a motivator. That is why it is so important for you to regularly record the number on the scale, your weight, each month. Also, you must tell your buddy. This process stays in place for the rest of your life! If I didn't think you needed constant support, I wouldn't tell you to follow this procedure. But you do, I do, everyone does who has a weight problem. You will be conscious forever that you will have to work to hold the line. Challenges are everywhere. It's not like you can hide food. You **have** to eat to stay well. For you to stay on the program, to stay fit, and to stay slim, it is necessary to stay motivated. When you look at your record and see what you have achieved, you will feel good. When you see that you are maintaining your ideal weight, you will feel terrific. When you look at your record and see that you gained weight, you will then know that you have had a slight misstep and you then spring into action. When you tell this to your buddy, you become accountable.

Every month you will get smarter as you study your pattern of fluctuation in weight loss and gain. By keeping notes on all weight gains, you will eventually learn what triggers your eating, or what situations need special attention. You are human, and we all have our ups and downs in life, and often these events are mirrored on the scale. With time and with practice, you will be able to hold your ideal weight.

Invest in yourself for the long haul. You are worthy of a great deal of personal study and introspection. Being overweight is a complex issue often with more than one cause or underlying factor. If your overeating is psychologically or emotionally charged, expect that it may take longer for you to reach your ideal weight than it would the person who is overweight because of a few bad habits or just enjoying food too much. I know that you are impatient to get the weight off, and you will. But give yourself the time that you need to do it right. As long as you are losing weight every month you are traveling in the right direction. When you seem to stall, it's because your body is fighting to hold on to the weight. Holding the line is also very important. Stay with the program and you will win.

It's your life

Even your best attempts to follow this program will be foiled if you do not truly love yourself. You must be willing to make a commitment to yourself and your health. You must think well enough of yourself to believe that you are worth it. Ultimately the answers to most of our problems can be solved from within. I cannot make you do anything. Only you can make yourself into the person you want to be. I can offer the blueprint, I can present the example, but you must take the action. The motivation comes from the small voice within that knows and loves you.

When we don't love ourselves, subconsciously we say, " I don't care. I'll eat myself sick." So many people, in fact, do exactly that. Chronic diseases are major causes of death, and often stem from a lifetime of self-abusive living habits. Is this our cry for help? Is this the way we get attention? Your body is the report card of how much you're hurting, and of how much you care about yourself.

You are responsible, by and large, for your own health within the parameters of predisposing genetic factors. Generally we realize how important our health is when it starts to disappear. People get caught by their bad habits. Look at the cancer patient who smokes. The overweight diabetic. The sedentary high blood pressure patient. These people thought perhaps that they were invulnerable. The truth is that the bad habits we allow into our lives can kill us. Do you care about the quality of your life? Are you good enough to deserve the self-esteem that comes from looking and feeling great?

While I have used the word "magic" to describe this eating plan, both you and I know that what I've given you is a hand trick to make balancing food groups and gauging portion sizes fun and easy. Any diet that takes you away from well-balanced eating is a fad diet. It's not good for the long-term and could damage your health even in the short-term. The most damage that the fad diet does, however, is to keep you from learning the principles of healthy well-balanced eating. It's a shortsighted view of weight loss. It may work for two weeks, but then where are you?

What I'm asking you to do is to change your life habits. Nothing less will do. And in small steps it is a manageable task. What you need is commitment and regular practice with a dose of self-discipline. They go hand in hand. Sometimes you may fight yourself. Remember every day is a new day on the MagicHand eating plan. Pick yourself up, start over again. People who quit when they fail will never be successful, but those who get back on track will achieve their goals.

Holding on

No matter how long it takes for you to reach your ideal weight, as long as you are on your way with consistent weight loss, <u>stick to the program</u>. You can "cheat" on this program, just as you could on any other. Don't sabotage yourself. The size of your palm is a very specific measure. If you don't believe me, you could measure it with a tape measure. Do not allow yourself to become careless with your "sizing". It's amazing how your palm can grow with loose interpretation.

In your past you may have been caught in a vicious cycle. If you've been sedentary, you've probably been so because you were overweight. Conversely, if you are overweight, pounds were added because you were sedentary. You may have been uninformed about good nutrition-- not knowing what good, healthy foods to include in your diet. And, some of us learned our bad habits in families where we had to eat what was on our plates whether hungry or not. Don't expect to extinguish every bad habit in a day. You are in training. New habits are developed with practice. Think about how long it took for you to brush your teeth without prompting. It's now a habit in your adult life. You wouldn't feel right without brushing your teeth now. That same thing can happen when you install this eating Plan in your life. You will never be able to look at food the same way again. You will immediately see palm portions. You will enjoy the results that come from counting.

Two in training

Adele is a spunky woman in her sixties, living alone in a retirement community. Her problem basically is that she likes to eat, especially peanuts and beer. When she came to me she was on blood pressure medication and carrying 170 pounds on her 5 ft. 1 in. frame. She was unhappy about taking blood pressure pills and wanted to improve her health. Her psychological attitude was wonderful and she had comparatively little stress in her life. But her mental image of herself as a fat lady was devastating. Her goal was to lose 10 pounds, to be 160 pounds. Included in her meditation were affirmations. She said to herself nightly, "I am 160 pounds. It is O.K. for me to weigh less." She began eating with her MagicHand and I asked her to call me when she reached her 160 pound weight sub-goal. Through a combination of meditation, fast walking and using her MagicHand she lost 10 pounds in 3 months. Her next sub-goal is 155 pounds. So far, so good.

Jane is a flight attendant for a major international airline. She has always had a problem keeping her weight under control. Flights take her to Lisbon, Paris, and Cairo, among other cities. She is juggling work stresses, international time changes, and disruptions in her eating patterns every time she flies. Needless to say, she is highly motivated to maintain a slim body weight since flight attendants are expected to present a trim, attractive appearance. She had already experienced just about every quick-loss diet in existence. She was really following the yo-yo method of weight loss. On one regimen she ended in the hospital after trying a liquid protein diet. Jane was in fairly good health and her main problem seemed to be her inability to stay with any one diet. She also had a "trick knee" limiting her capability for exercise. She started this Plan and was delighted that her measurer, her hand, was always with her. It made eating pre-packaged flight meals easy to use. She found time to fast-walk almost every day when the weather was good. She had failed to plan ahead with a contingency plan for a cold weather activity so she "lost" three weeks of physical play while she tried to decide what else she could do. It broke the momentum, but with an upcoming wedding to motivate her, she reached her ideal weight in short order. The real challenge came after the wedding when she slipped back to her old eating habits. Then she returned to MagicHand eating proving to herself that she simply cannot be in control of her weight, without controlling her portion sizes.

These stories illustrate that we are all human and need to keep the motivation to stay slim to propel us forward. What is **your** reason for wanting to stay slim? The best reason you could give me is that you want to feel good about yourself and be the best, healthiest "you" there is. Many women want to become slender in order to attract men or even to stay fat to keep men away. Some people want to become trim to get a job or to be fat to decrease their chances of being hired. Yet others want to be slim only for their wedding pictures and plan on freely indulging the rest of their married life. Most people are motivated to lose weight for some reason: their doctor has told them to, they are getting married, or perhaps they want to look good in a swim suit. People are motivated to fail at losing weight also for some reason: not to be attractive, to have a "problem", or perhaps with larger size-- gain "authority" to psychologically compensate for the areas in their lives that might be deficient.

Become healthy and slim for yourself, for the pleasure it will bring you, and then nothing can threaten your determination and motivation to win. Although I have consistently emphasized the importance of correct body weight, remember, that as you become more fit, and muscle tissue starts to replace fat tissue, some weight gain is possible.

Occasionally take your measurements too. Keep a pair of "target slacks" in your closet and look at yourself. If you start to gain weight and the slacks look better, you'll know the extra weight is due to firmer muscle.

This Plan is designed for people who want to lose weight and maintain that loss in a healthy manner. It is also necessary to accept the fact that to effect this change you must permanently live a life of controlled eating. You may know people who can eat anything and not gain weight, but if you were one of them, you would not be reading this book. So, let's make our pact.

Are we having fun yet?
A sense of humor and losing weight often don't seem to go together. This program should be fun. Think of it as a game. You against excess food. Move the magnets on your MagicHand diagram that you may have posted on your refrigerator as if you were winning at checkers or backgammon.
(Or use another way to count chits. See *Appendix D*.)

Every day that you have successfully stayed within or completed all the palm and thumb portions in the food groups, you've won. (You know you'll be paying a penalty if you go over the allotted chits.) Every day it's a new game.

Take a look at your hand again. It's a simple little tool that can work for you.

You'll never have to count calories, fat grams or weigh foods again. Remember the slogan: **"My Fingers Count Portions Offering Variety."** From pinky to thumb you can remember the food groups: **M**ilk & Dairy, **F**ruit, **C**arbohydrate, **P**rotein and **O**ils. These are the players in the game and you must include 3 of each every day. Vegetables are unlimited. A total of 12 palm portions and 3 thumbs a day! Keep hydrated with water.

Consider yourself in training with the rest of your life to practice.
Go for it!

Hand in hand

You want to lose weight. You want to stay at your ideal weight for the rest of your life. Do we know what you want? So, let's begin. Commit to this Plan for the next 3 weeks. In that time you will break old habits and learn how to eat properly. I am asking you to devote the next 3 weeks, the next 21 days of your life, to experience what healthy eating is like, and to witness your body take new shape. Count the days on your calendar.

After 21 days, you decide if you want to go back to your old way of eating and weight gain. I think you will find that you are happier and healthier at the end of this period than ever. I want you to prove to yourself that you can do it, and that you can look forward to a lifetime of healthy eating. This investment in a future full of good health and happiness is worth the effort. The initial 3-week period, getting started, is the first big step. To keep yourself motivated study one of the nine Points each week. If you have friends who want to lose weight, form a group and meet weekly to discuss each focus point. (See *Appendix C*). You will find that you learn from others and that their support will keep you going. After you have gone through all nine focus Points, you should be well practiced in the principles of the program. At the end of these 3 weeks, ask yourself, "What are the results?" If you have lost weight, and you have found the program livable make an even deeper commitment to keeping it in place. You now know if it works for you. Can we shake hands on that? If after 21 days of consistently using your MagicHand you have experienced more normal healthy eating, and you have lost weight, and you feel good, vow that you will **commit** to keeping this Plan in place for **the rest of your life**.

I believe that your new pattern of eating will be so rewarding that you will be motivated to maintain your results. Consider yourself as if in training for the Olympics-- but instead this is a training for life. Like any artist or athlete you will always be perfecting your skills and continuing to learn.

If you lose weight, and then go back to your old way of eating, you can expect what? To gain back the weight you lost. Don't do it. Be good to yourself. Love yourself well.

Take away message: To keep your weight under control follow this program — adopt healthy habits for life.

Now, listen...
the sound of two hands clapping.

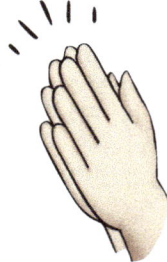

PRACTICE

The mission of the dr.Anne Association is to promote healthy well-balanced eating for weight control and to make it easy and fun. And to provide Practice Circles for support.

Most people need support when changing habits. To stay motivated we strongly recommend that you participate in an on-going Practice Circle. If you would like to create your own Circle see Appendix C for details.

The purpose of this Practice is to provide useful self-help exercises to be completed in the privacy of your own home or in a Circle group setting. By writing down your answers you can help yourself become clear about where you stand on psychological, physical, and practical issues. This process may force you to think about your lifestyle and what is good for you. Make sure to write down your answers to the questions posed since this very act solidifies your words and thoughts.

You can't help someone who doesn't want to help himself.
Guidance for the changes you are willing to make. Practice for life.

Start

dr. Anne plan

• Point 1 Practice

1

Getting to know your FINGER FOODS

What foods do I really like to eat? List those foods and identify the food group in which they belong: (Milk&Dairy, Fruit, Carbohydrate, Protein, Oils/Fats & Sweets, or Vegetables) *See Appendix E for Food Groups.* After the food indicate with an "X" if it is a trigger food for you, that is, once you have one you can't stop having another.

Example: *ice cream*   Trigger?   Food group: *Milk & Dairy*

_____   _____   _____

_____   _____   _____

_____   _____   _____

_____   _____   _____

_____   _____   _____

_____   _____   _____

_____   _____   _____

_____   _____   _____

_____   _____   _____

_____   _____   _____

How would you measure the portion size for each one listed?

_____

Some foods may be a combination of different foods (like pizza) so decide how you might wish to categorize the food. In this case, for example, you could call pizza a "Carbohydrate" or a "Milk" or even a "Protein". You could list it under one or all three. In actual practice you will be counting your palm-size portion in one of these food groups, but when foods are in combination there is some flexibility.

95

Did you have at least one favorite food that was in each of the six food groups? If not, you might want to take another look at Seeing Fingers Appendix E. Find the foods in each food group that you like and add them to your list to create your own special menus.

Designing your daily menu

To practice eating the MagicHand way, design your own menu. Custom tailor each day so that you include foods from each of the food groups and count the number of palm-portion chits. Use the foods you previously listed in each of the food groups to create a menu that you'll enjoy eating. If you are better at following a structured menu plan, repeat this process for the next 7 days. Then make believe that you are on a "diet"-- and this is what you have to eat. Thereafter you are the master who can create and follow well-balanced menus. Using your palm-portions you will keep your weight under control long-term. Go for it!

My Menu

Meal	Food Group Item	Palm/thumb portion
Breakfast (Time)		
Snack:		
Lunch: (Time)		
Snack:		
Dinner: (Time)		

Number of Palm-portions:_____   **Number** of Thumb-portions:_____

For Practice Circle discussion:

What foods do I really like to eat? How would I measure the portion-size? In what food group or groups does it belong?

_____

_____

Wave your wand!

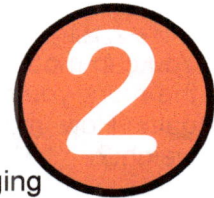

● Point 2 Practice

2

After you have reached your ideal weight, you can start the challenging process of maintaining that weight. Remember your weight range. If you ever go two pounds over your ideal weight you must return to strictly adhering to the food groups and portion controls of your MagicHand.

How far can you deviate? You could simply bring back some foods you enjoy that you know are calorie-dense still keeping them in palm-portions. You will discover for yourself how far you can deviate without gaining weight through a process of trial and error. If you start to gain weight, vow to return to the rules of your MagicHand. Always stay conscious and continue eating in palm portions. This is a forever llife plan. Your old ways of eating resulted in disaster! Do not think you're on holiday because you achieved your ideal weight and interpret that accomplishment as a signal that you can return to your old eating habits. You must keep the MagicHand in place. Never let it go.

Consider for a moment if there are any favorite foods that you don't eat in order to lose weight. List those foods in the left column. What food group? How would you serve that food in a palm or thumb portion?

Favorite Food.	Food Group.	Palm/thumb portion
_____ . _____		_____
_____ . _____		_____
_____ . _____		_____

Think about your favorite foods. How could you "stretch" those portions?
Are there any foods you could "stretch" by adding Vegetables?

What food group(s) do I want to eat the most?

_____   _____

What food group(s) do I like the least or have difficulty getting into my diet?

_____

Could I meet the nutritional benefit of that food group(s) I don't like in some other way?

How?

_____

_____

You can modify your MagicHand by trading the chits from one food group to another. But the more you deviate, the less balanced the diet, and perhaps the more likely for weight gain. How many food group "trades" do you think you could make without gaining weight?

_____

For Practice Circle discussion:

Did you discover any ways to "stretch" your favorite foods with vegetables? If so, how?

_____

_____

Are there any food preparation tricks you use to make healthful desserts?

_____

_____

What has been the most challenging problem for you to overcome with food preparation?

_____

_____

_____

Food Preparation Ideas:

Variety is the spice of life!

● Point 3 Practice

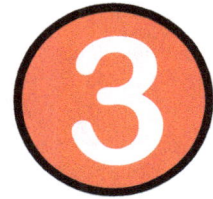

3

Eating challenges

How can I *hand*le eating away from home? Fortuantely you can plan ahead to meet the challenges of restaurant dining, house parties, holidays and travel. In this section we will provide training for how you can order from a restaurant menu.

Use the sample menu provided on the next page, or better yet, study the menu from one of your local restaurants. In all situations you will be able to use your MagicHand, but it takes practice.

Imagine you are with a group of friends and you all decide to go out to eat dinner. You still have 4 palm portions and 1 thumb oil remaining for the day. How will you order? What will you eat?

There is more than one correct answer.
Look at the next page and pretend you are ordering now. Say: "I will have...

_____

_____
_____".

It might be helpful to look at the dessert menu first so that you will know how many chits you have left for the meal.
How you will use your chits? Name the food. My:

Milk palm-portion is for _____

Fruit palm-portion is for _____

Carbohydrate palm-portion is for_____

Protein palm-portion is for _____

Oil/fat thumb-portion is for _____

Vegetables are: _____

Now imagine that you receive the order and visualize the food in front of you. How large are each of the portions? Describe. To keep to palm portion sizes, what food will be left on your plate?

_____

FULLY'S

APPETIZERS

Peel and eat shrimp...   Crab stuffed mushrooms......
Calamari strips............   Sautéed mushrooms...........
Steamed artichoke..........   Chicken fingers.............

SALADS

Caesar salad..............   Chicken Caesar.............
(served with garlic bread)

PRIME RIB-STEAKS-RIBS

All dinner entrees served with your choice of
homemade French onion soup or a garden salad, fresh baked bread and your choice of a baked potato,
French fries, Rice pilaf or Spanish rice. Have an enjoyable evening.

Fully's prime rib (full cut)...............................
Fully's prime rib (half-cut).........................
Porterhouse..
Filet Mignon...
New York Steak..

SHELLFISH, FISH & CHICKEN

Australian lobster- 1 tail...............................
Alaskan King crab.......................................
Shrimp scampi...
Breast of chicken   (choice of teriyaki or BBQ sauce).........
Fresh fish of the day   (white wine & lemon or garlic butter).

DESSERTS

Ice cream pie..............   New York cheesecake.......

BEVERAGES

Coffee, tea ....   Milk, buttermilk...........

What will you doggie bag?_____

If you decided to have dessert, what palm portion(s) if any, will you need to trade?

_____

What dessert will you order?_____

Is it likely to come in a palm portion size?_____

Party pushers

Saying no to food is something most of us have not learned. We must learn the secrets of the slim people, and again it takes practice

There are people called "pushers". At a party they will say, "Have another piece." At dinner they will say, "You must have seconds."

Because of pushers you will need to learn how to become a "slim-sayer". The slim-sayer knows what to say to counter the pusher. The pusher considers the person on a diet to be a challenge. So, never tell the pusher you are watching how much you eat. Think of the phrases that thin people say. If you can, with another person, each trade roles, as a "pusher" and "slim-sayer", in the following exercise.

For Practice Circle participation:

Play this "game" with a partner. Imagine you are at a relative's home. A feast is on the table. Everyone has brought a "special" dish. It is the pusher's job to get you to have more food. It is the slim-sayer's job to politely decline.

Supply the "pusher" statement:

_____

_____

Supply the "slim-sayer" response:

_____

_____

Now trade places with your partner and do the same exercise again. You can play this game as long as you like. Try to find the responses that feel comfortable to you. And remember even if someone pushes something on your plate, you don't have to eat it.

No Chit Days

Your job has been to learn how to use your MagicHand for every day eating and a lifetime of staying slim. But every job has some vacation time built in. Each day you start with 12 palm portion chits and 3 thumb portion chits. The program is absolutely livable. But, there are some times when you would really like **not** to count chits. Thanksgiving, for example, might be one day. On the program you are permitted nine days a year where you do not need to count chits. These are no-chits days and you should decide ahead of time what days they will be. This does not mean that you gorge yourself on the day; it just means you don't have to count or worry about palm portion eating. In other words, you can have that birthday, eat as much of what you want, and still stay on the program.

Go through the months of the year and think of the special occasions or holidays when you would like **not** to count chits. Remember that the reason you are monitoring your food intake is because you have a tendency to gain weight when left to your own devices. So, it can't be that every day is a no-chit day!

Think of the days during the year that are special days for you that might include a festive eating celebration. If you have more than nine special days, cut back some days. If you have less than nine, be aware that you then have some "floating days" to use some other time. Our year starts in January, so let's begin.

Next to the month place the date of the occasion or name the holiday when you would like a no-chit day. Select nine days over the year.

Your party planner for the year:
You have 9 no-chit days each year

Month	Date	Month	Date
January		July	
February		August	
March		September	
April		October	
May		November	
June		December	

If you have any days left over they are: floating days=____

What days will you not be counting chits? Mark these days on your calendar as "No-chit days". I hope you will find as I have, that even on your no-chit days, because you have been trained in how to eat during the year, you still think in palm portions. Nevertheless it's nice to have a break once in a while, and it's also nice to get back to counting chits since we know it brings us the reward of good health and appearance

Minefields ahead!

102

dr. Anne plan

● Point 4 Practice

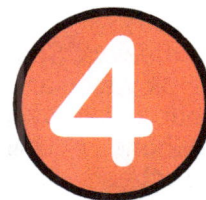

4

Recording your numbers

Let's establish your health baseline according to some physical measurements.

Plan to update and review these measures every year as part of your own physical evaluation. As you lose weight you will see these measures improve.

Do this at home: the 'Mirror Test'

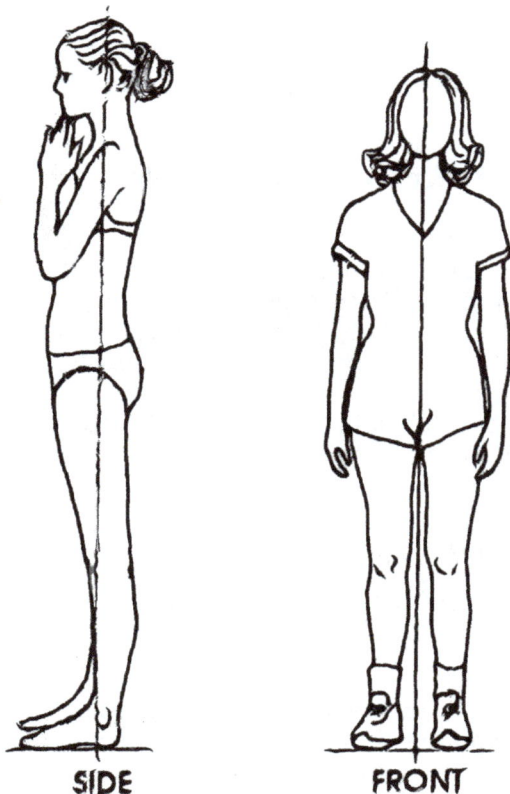

SIDE   FRONT

(This may take courage, but do it anyway.) Stand in front of a full-length mirror without any clothes and take a good look. Point your toes forward and observe your body shape. Imagine a line going lengthwise through the center of your body. Are you lopsided? Standing straight? Now turn sideways. Squeeze your buttocks and pull in your "stomach" abdominal muscles.

Do this now: While seated, place your hands on your mid-section and find your abdominal muscles. Can you locate them? While exhaling, try to pull them in. Breathe out and tighten your abdominals.

Notice any difference? Any thoughts about your body? _____

103

Homework Special Assignment: Now, take the "pulse test". This is an indicator of your cardiovascular health. While you are lying in bed-- before you arise in the morning-- find your pulse by placing your middle fingers on the side of the neck just under your jawbone. Using the second hand on your watch or timer, count the number of heartbeats you feel in 15 seconds. Then multiply this number by 4 to get the number of heartbeats in a minute (60 seconds). Repeat this procedure until you get a consistent number. A good/average pulse rate is considered 80 heartbeats per minute. More than that and you are probably out of condition!

15 second pulse rate is: _____ X 4 = _____ beats per minute.

A field trip! Your Medical records: If you have results from a recent blood test or physical exam, keep this information as a permanent record and store it in a folder, binder or on your computer.

It would be wise to get a blood test yearly and to keep these records yourself as reference. These results will act as personal health "markers". Look for changes in your own baseline blood test values to indicate changes in your health status. Keep in mind that blood test reference values sometimes will change either in accordance with new research or the laboratory used. Dr. George Z. Williams, a noted pathologist, advised to keep your own "when in good health" blood test values as your gold standard reference. Each body is different and tests are based on averages. What's important is to watch for changes in yourself and then determine if the direction in blood test value is positive or negative. I suggest not to rush into medicating if lifestyle change might work first. Retesting every year is prudent.

The right range numbers
Your weight is the number that registers on the scale. The goal is to maintain your ideal weight-- to see that number register as the best weight for your body design. If you are not sure what the best or ideal healthy weight is for yourself, here is a simple formula you can use:

For women, start with 100 lbs. for five feet of height. For every inch over five feet add 5 pounds. For example, if you are 5 feet 4 inches in height, you should weigh 100 lbs. + 20 lbs.= 120 pounds assuming an average or medium frame body build.

For men, start with 106 lbs. for five feet of height. For every inch over five feet add 6 pounds. Making this more complicated, let's say you are a 6' 3 1/2" man, then your ideal weight according to this formula, given a medium frame, would be 106 + (15.5 in. X 6 lbs.) or 93 = 199 pounds. But, assuming you are large boned, you would then add 10%, for an "ideal weight" of (199 + 19.9) = 218.9 or, rounding off, 219 pounds.

Here is a quick and easy way to determine if you are "small-boned" or "large-boned". Measure the circumference of your non-dominant wrist at its smallest part by wrapping the thumb and middle finger of the other hand around it.

You are small-boned if your thumb and middle finger overlap. You are large-boned if the fingers don't touch. If the fingers just touch you are medium framed.

If you are small-boned <u>subtract</u> 10% from your answer. If you are large-boned <u>add</u> 10% to your answer. (Remember these estimates are approximate and by no means the last word on what you should weigh. Muscle tissue weighs more than fat tissue so if you are very muscular this estimate might be low and conversely, if you have a lot of fat tissue and little muscle, this estimate might be too high.)

Guideline to my "ideal" weight:

For women: 100 lbs. + _____ = _____
        (add or subtract 10%)=_____

For men: 106 lbs. + _____ = _____
        (add or subtract 10%)=_____

           My "ideal" weight according to this formula is:_____

I agree with this?   YES   or   NO   Why? _____

Make sure you do this now!
The "ideal" weight I have set for myself is: _____

My "ideal weight range" is established by subtracting and adding two pounds to my "ideal" weight. Write down your ideal weight range from low to high with the ideal weight in the middle. Circle or underline your ideal weight.
My Ideal Weight Range is :

_____   _____   _____
Low -2   Ideal   +2 High

        My present weight is: _____   Date:_____

            Every **month** I will report my weight to my buddy.
            My buddy is:

            _____

            Every **month** I will record my weight.
            My monthly recording date is:_____

105

dr. Anne plan
Find an index card or use the one below. Tape the card inside your bath medicine cabinet or a closet door.
Or keep track on a spreadsheet.

Write your name and weight information on the top line of the card.

On the top line: (your name)   -2 ⟨ Ideal Weight ⟩ +2   Year:

Date (Day)	Weight		Note:

For Practice Circle Discussion:
How can I best take care of my health? (Answer this question for yourself first.)

_____

How healthy am I? What health benefit will I get from losing weight? (Answer this

question for yourself first.)_____

_____

What will I use to keep a record of my weight? An index card? File on my computer?

_____

You're on your way!

● Point 5 Practice

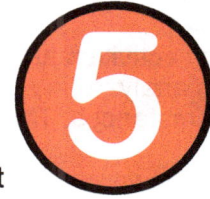

5

How much should I exercise?

You must determine for yourself the physical play activities you want to pursue. The objective is to find pleasure or joy in what you select.

Before we discuss what is feasible, let's take a look at a number of physical play activities. Without thinking of the exercise benefits of any these activities, go through the list and check the ones that you "like" or for some reason, appeal to you. This list includes over fifty activities enjoyable to a great many people. Of course, there are more, so add any others that you might like as well. From this list select those activities that excite you. Don't concern yourself now with any limitations you may have in pursuing the activity. (I know if you live in Florida you won't go snow skiing every day.) Never mind. Simply go through the list and quickly place a check mark next to your favorite activities or those you'd like to do.

aerobic dancing	gardening	scuba/skin diving
Aikido/Tai chi	golf	shuffleboard
archery	gymnastics	skateboarding
badminton	handball	skiing/ downhill/X-C
ballet	hiking/backpacking	snowboarding
baseball/softball	hockey/ field/ice	snowshoeing
basketball	horseback riding	soccer
bicycling	ice/figure skating	spinning
bocce ball	judo/karate	square dancing
boogieboard	kayaking	squash
bowling	lacrosse	surfing/board/wind
boxing/wrestling	mtn. climbing	swimming
caisthenics	paddle ball	table tennis
canoeing	pickleballi	tap dancing
cricket	polo	tennis
dancing/ ballroom	raquetball	trampoline/mini
diving	roller skating	treadmill
fencing	rope skipping	volleyball
fitness trail	rowing	walking
flexibility exercises	rugby	water skiing
football/touch	running/jogging	weight lifting
frisbee	sailing/yachting	Yoga

Many activities are only enjoyable if the weather is good, but we can plan around that. Let's analyze and plan a physical play program designed especially for you and your life circumstances. This will become the overall picture of your physical play program.

Write down your favorite sports or outdoor activities: (at least one for each season).

Summer _____

Fall _____

Winter _____

Spring _____

What do you need to get started now? (Equipment, facilities, etc.)

_____

_____

What would be an alternative 'physical play' if it rains, or your practice partner doesn't show up, or you are traveling or something else happens?

_____

_____

When and where will you practice your 'pelvic tilt'?

_____

Your exercise prescription
You need to get started. And the time is now. What is the season now? Let's look at your list again. Select a favorite activity that would be appropriate for this season. Of all the convenient, fun, possible physical play activities on your list, which one will you select to start?

Exercise Prescription

Season: _____

Main play activity:_____

Alternatives/Back-up:_____

_____

Place: _____

How often: _____

What length of time:_____

For Practice Circle participation:
Knowing how to walk properly and hold your body is a basic first step to any physical activity. With someone seated across the room watching you, walk five steps forward. Are your feet straight? Do you walk as if on a straight line or are your toes pointing out or in? Is your body aligned?

For Practice Circle discussion:
Do you want to set aside a specific amount of time (at least 30 minutes) during the day for physical play or would you rather accumulate times of activity (at least 30 minutes) throughout the day. What would be easier for you?

_____

Do you have any obstacles right now to starting your physical activity? If so, what are they? How can they be overcome?

_____

_____

Any exercise is better than no exercise!

● Point 6 Practice

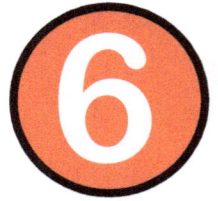

How can I find the time to stay healthy?
Let's look at a day in your life. Using the clock diagram below describe
your own "typical" day, from the time you arise until the time you go to bed. (If you're
employed pick a normal work day.) Identify blocks of time by drawing a line from the
center of the clock to the outside perimeter. Inside each pie-shaped block of time write
in the activity that occurs in that time period for your "typical" day. Do this in light pencil.

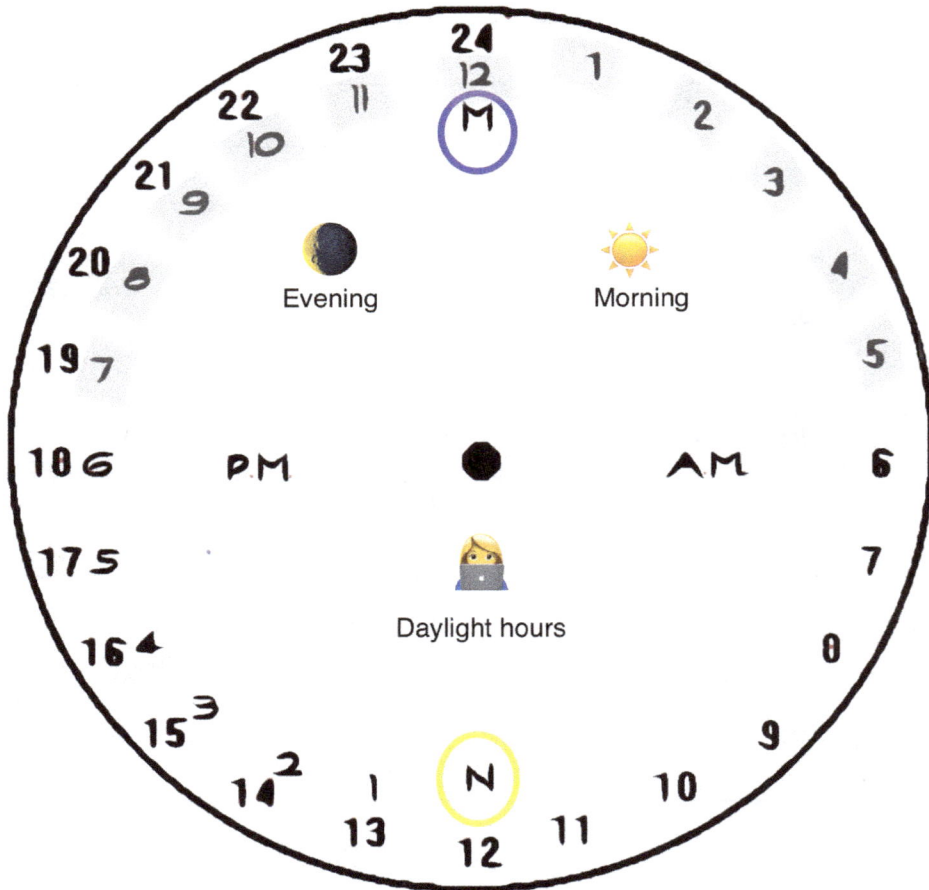

Evening

Morning

P.M

AM

Daylight hours

Right now, does your day include some time for eating regular meals, for physical play or
exercise, and for meditation?

If not, let's find some time to include these activities.   Study your day and determine when you might include the practices you need to stay healthy. For example, you could include physical exercise before breakfast in the morning, perhaps before lunch, before dinner or before bedtime. Keep in mind the physical play activity you have selected for this season.

Could you meditate after lunch or after dinner or before bedtime? When are your opportunities for exercise or physical play? When could you take 20 minutes for meditation? To feel good, how many hours of sleep do you require?

Using a pen or colored marker now draw in the hours on that clock diagram to show your health practice times.

- (1) First draw in the time for eating meals
- (2) then the time(s) that you will exercise, and
- (3) a time for meditation
- After these priorities, you can now add the other activities that normally consume your day.

For Practice Circle discussion:
Are others in my life robbing me of time?   If so, what could I do differently to put my needs first? State one concrete action.

_____

_____

At present do I make time to eat regular meals?

_____

At present do I make time to meditate or reflect quietly for about 20 minutes each day?

_____

At present do I make time for a regular physical play exercise activity?

_____

What would I have to do to get the time I need to stay healthy? State one concrete action you could take immediately to free twenty minutes in your day.

_____

_____

"It is worthy to perform the present duty well and without failure; do not seek to avoid or postpone it till tomorrow. By acting now one can have a good day."   — *Bukkyo Dendo Kyokai*

It's worth your time!

dr. Anne plan

● Point 7 Practice

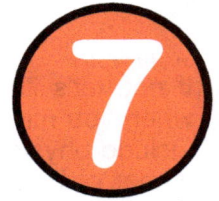

How do my mind and body interact?
Some part of you must decide that you deserve to become the person you want to be both physically and psychologically. Are you fighting yourself? Your feelings may be controlling your eating behavior. We will explore some of those feelings in this Practice section. It is time for you to take charge of those emotions.

Is there something about my body that I do not like? If so, what?

_____

Would losing weight make it better?

_____

What is it about my body that I do like?

_____

Visualize your body at your ideal weight. See this as your achievable goal. Whenever you think about your body or look at yourself in the mirror see yourself at your ideal weight or if you have a lot of weight to lose, just see yourself with five pounds less.

A mental exercise
Look at yourself as you are right now. Keep taking off five pounds until you visually reach your ideal weight. Every time you take off five pounds ask yourself, "How do I feel?" Was that weight serving any purpose? If not, release that fat visually. Let it go. Say to yourself: "I am on my way to my ideal weight." And be happy. Put a smile on your face. Know that you can achieve and maintain your ideal weight goal for a lifetime.

Very important
Your feelings are very important and will either assist you or sabotage you as you get closer to your ideal weight. Not only must you stay with the Plan, but you must also become keenly aware of the times when you overeat or binge or simply stuff yourself. Do not consider these events as failures-- they are learning opportunities crucial to your eventual success! You might wish to keep a journal and record the date, precipitating event, your feelings, your reaction, and upon reflection, what you could do other than eating to handle your emotions.

Take charge
If you gain weight during a month, there is a reason why. Whenever you see an increase in weight on your monthly record, describe in one or two words on the same line what event or circumstance might be responsible under the heading "Note". Then determine what you could do differently or if there is an emotional factor that deserves your introspection. For example, you might have gained weight because of not counting palm portions at your sister's birthday party, or because of an emotional upset from an ex-spouse's visit, or simply from counting ice cream in your Milk food group too many times. Determine how you will handle these situations and your use of food the next time to prevent weight gain. If you notice that every time your ex-spouse visits you gain

weight because of an eating binge try to identify the feeling (anger?) and attempt either through your own self-talk or with a counselor to resolve the hurt. Get in control.

Overeating style
How would you describe your weight-gain eating style?

Are you a High Intake Appestat eater?_____

Are you a Food Trigger Binger?_____

Are you a Stuffing Feelings Eater?_____

A combination?_____

Think back to a time when you simply ate too much, or had a binge eating episode, or just kept stuffing yourself with food. Can you remember what happened or how you were feeling? Describe.

_____

_____

_____

Now take this feeling(s) and think of another action you could take (besides eating) that would make you feel better or could help you to release the emotion?   Complete the sentence:

When I am feeling_____I could_____.

When I am feeling_____I could_____.

When I am feeling_____I could_____.

For Practice Circle discussion:
Try to identify the mood you are in right now. Say "I'm feeling_____."
Someone in the group volunteer to tell a short funny story and no matter how funny or unfunny it is, everyone must laugh with a "ho,ho,ho". Go ahead.

Now, how are you feeling? Did your mood change? Do you have the power to change how you're feeling?

_____

_____

Feel the feeling!

• Point 8 Practice

8

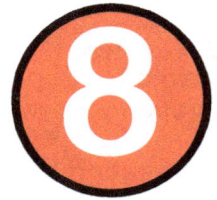

What is "food" for my soul?
1. Name five activities that you really enjoy doing.

_____

_____

_____

_____

2. If you haven't already, select one of the above that you can incorporate into your life now. How can you put this activity into your life on a regular basis?

_____

_____

3. Name one thing that you haven't done in a long time that really nurtures or pampers you

_____

What would have to happen for you to enjoy this now?

_____

For stress reduction practice slow breathing
One of the best things you can do for yourself to relieve distress is to practice abdominal breathing. Take long deep breaths that fully distend your rib cage and abdomen; then exhale slowly through your mouth. When you are about to face a tense situation remember to pause and take at least three deep breaths. It may not solve the problem but it will help you to take care of yourself.

Practice slow breathing whenever you want to calm yourself or in preparation for and during meditation.

Try this exercise right now. Stand straight.   Place one hand against the small of your back and the other on your abdomen. Breathe in slowly, as if you are filling a tank and allow your midsection to expand. Your hand should feel some movement.   (If your shoulders move this is a sign of incorrect breathing.)   As you exhale tighten the abdominal muscles and release the air through your mouth blowing the stress away. Tilt your mid-section towards your back hand. When doing this exercise or any other where muscles are tightened and released, remember that the muscle is always tightened on the exhale (push the air out) and the muscle is relaxed on the inhale (fill up).

So, breathe in and fill the abdomen- relax the muscles.

Breathe out and tighten the abdomen- tighten the pelvic muscles. To relieve stress and feel better practice abdominal breathing. (Note: You will automatically breathe abdominally if you do this exercise while lying with your back flat on the floor.)

For Practice Circle participation:

If you have never meditated or have never consciously allotted a time to be quiet, you can now experience this silence. You will need a comfortable chair to sit in. Place your feet on the floor and sit straight. If you'd like, remove your shoes. With a timer allow yourself ten minutes of silence. Close your eyes and continue to breathe deeply. Soft restful music can play in the background. Some people may giggle at first-- that's okay, or you might feel awkward with others around. Calm down, relax, breathe deeply and just do it. Sit quietly for ten minutes and push your thoughts away. Mainly concentrate on your breathing. It takes much practice to push all thoughts out of your mind so if they come, gently let them go, and push them away. See if you can simply "be" sitting on your chair in tune with the rhythm of your own breathing. During this meditation when you feel you are really relaxed, almost in a semi-sleep state, you may wish to imagine yourself losing five pounds. Keep taking five pounds off of your body and seeing yourself at a reduced weight until you reach your ideal weight. Repeat an affirmation: "I am now at my ideal body weight of _____." As the pounds leave and you see yourself slimmer, let go of the weight you no longer want or need. Send it away.
Are you comfortable? Are you ready? Silence begin.

For Practice Circle discussion:

The experience of ten minutes of silence for some people is unsettling because disturbing thoughts that have been pushed down can surface. Eventually you will be able to resolve and push away recurring thoughts. Remember that the silence of meditation is healing. Your goal is to meditate each day for twenty minutes. This experience shows how long just ten minutes of silence feels, and how restful it can be. Some people awaken from meditation feeling as if they have been on a restful "vacation".

What was your experience in these moments of silence?

_____

_____

When could you find the time to meditate on a daily basis?

_____

Every day's a new day!

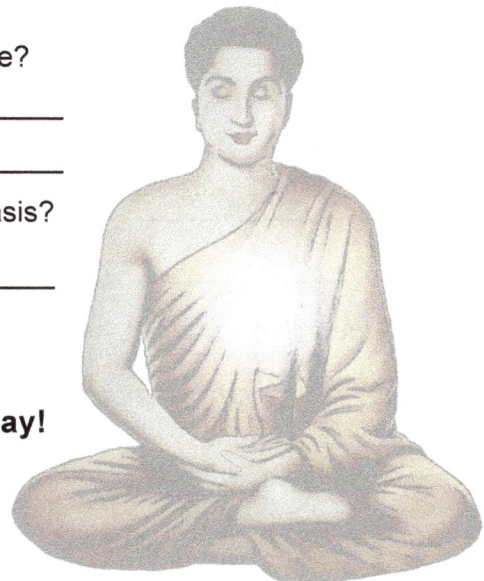

115

● Point 9 Practice

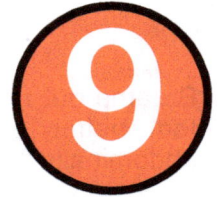

9

A thumbnail sketch
You have been offered a hand-trick for keeping your weight under control. What you need to do is learn all the food groups that the fingers of your hand represent and understand that the finger food groups above the palm of your hand are measured in palm portion sizes. Your thumb measure is used for fats and oils and concentrated sugars. You are allowed twelve palm and three thumb portions a day. Vegetables are unlimited. Every day is a new day. If for some reason you do not consume all of your chits they are not saved for the next day. Also if you go over your allotted chits one day, you do not hold back chits on the next day. Every day you get fifteen chits, twelve palms and three thumbs. So, every day is a new day with your MagicHand.

To stay motivated on this program for the rest of your life requires some self-knowledge. The following questions may not be easy to answer, but will help you discover what is really behind your desire for weight loss and control.

What are your reasons for losing weight? Why do you want to lose weight? Are these good enough reasons for a lifetime? (List your reasons).

_____

_____

Can you picture yourself at your ideal weight?   What difference will maintaining your ideal weight make in your life?

_____

_____

_____

Are there any obstacles? Is there anything holding you back from achieving your ideal weight?

_____

_____

Are you able to say that you love yourself enough to invest in your own well-being?

_____

The magic wand
The answers to the previous questions may make the difference between success and failure. For you to be successful you must stay with the program. Every day think of how

nice it will be to fit into your ideal size clothes. You can mentally have that pleasure now while your body catches up with the image you have created.

We are all motivated by the principles of pleasure and pain. And we can approach weight loss through a positive or negative avenue or a combination of both. To be clear about your own reasons for controlling your weight think about what is truly supporting your desire. If we are in pain, physically or psychologically, because of being overweight, we will want to stop the pain-- to do something about our condition. If we are in pleasure and joy about ourselves, our feelings of good self-worth and self-esteem will direct us to take care of our bodies.

Is your desire for weight control to eliminate the pain of being overweight? If so, describe this pain.

_____

_____

Is your desire for weight control to acknowledge a love for yourself by taking care of your body? If so, what will be the benefit?

_____

_____

Palm and thumb counters
Many people on this Plan have thought of creative ways to keep count of their 12 palm and 3 thumb daily portions. For example, some people use paper tear-offs to count their chits, others use a pencil check mark in their check registers, and some move coins from one pocket to another to count chits. Another has used clothespins. The most graphic presentation is to see your own hand on paper and to count your chits on the food group fingers each day.

For Practice Circle discussion:
What are you using to count chits? _____

Are you strictly following the program or using modifications? Explain.

_____

Once you have lost your weight, would you be tempted to go back to your old patterns of eating? If so, how can you motivate yourself to stay with the program?

_____

_____

Can you commit to living this way the rest of your life to maintain your ideal weight?

_____

Open Sesame!

117

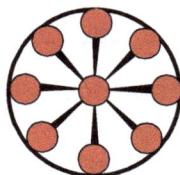

Appendices

A MagicHand Equivalent Measure
B MagicHand Cookery
C Practice Circles for Support
D MagicHand Chits Page
E Seeing Fingers on your MagicHand

Appendix A

MagicHand EQUIVALENT MEASURES

MagicHand	STANDARD

For Milk & Dairy, Fruit, Carbohydrates and Proteins:

1 Palm portion, spooned or soft food =	2-3. T.
1 Palm portion, liquid=	1/4-1/2 cup
1 Palm portion that's rounded =	1/4-1/2 cup
1 Palm portion, Thumb thick=	1-4 oz.

For Oils & Fats:

1 Thumb joint, solid=	1 t.
1 Thumb joint, semi-soft=	1 t.
1 Thumb of oil (if watered down/liquid)=	1 T.

For Vegetables:
Unmeasured/ Unlimited

For Sauces, Gravies, Syrups, Stews, Casseroles, Mixed Beverages, Fast Foods, Exotic Desserts, Preserves, Candy, and Other unidentified foods:

1 Palm portion, (sugar/fat laden) liquid, soft or spooned=	2-3 T.
1 Palm portion,liquid, rounded,held or cut=	1/4-1/2 cup or 1-4 oz.
1 Thumb (fat/sugar laden) liquid or spooned=	1 T.
1 Thumb (fat/sugar laden) watered down=	1 T.
1 Thumb-joint (fat/sugar laden) solid, hard or semi-soft=	1 t.

When in doubt: Important

Each chit portion ideally should be no more than 100 calories. The default for a cupped palm is 1/3 cup. The less fat and sugar in a palm portion, the fewer the calories. The more fiber in a palm portion, the healthier. MagicHand measures vary due to differences in hand size. STANDARD measures are precise. The hand measure is not perfect, but it works!

Appendix B

MagicHand COOKERY

SOUP, SALAD AND SUCH	Food Group

FRESH VEGETABLE BORSCH SOUP

1/4 chopped onion	V
1 cup shredded green cabbage	V
1 cup fresh beets, peeled and diced	V
1/2 carrot, shredded	V
2 1/4 cups tomato/vegetable juice	V
1/2 tomato chopped	V
1 T. lemon juice	free
1 T. soy sauce (optional)	free
1 t. fresh parsley, chopped	V
1/4 t. dill weed.	V
1 T. plain yogurt	M

Add onion, beets, cabbage, and carrot to the tomato juice in large saucepan or kettle. Bring to a boil, cover and simmer for 20 minutes. Add tomato, lemon juice and herbs. Simmer for another 15 minutes. For one serving, top with a dollop (1 T.) of yogurt.
1 serving= 1/2 Milk chit, Unlimited Vegetable

PITA POCKET MEAL

1 pita bread pocket sandwich	C
1/2 cup alfalfa sprouts	V
1 slice natural low-fat cheese (2 oz.)	M
4 oz. fish or chicken	P
1 t. mayonnaise	O
1 t. mustard	free

Spread mayonnaise and mustard inside pita bread. Stuff with cheese and fish or chicken, and sprouts. Makes 1 serving.
1 serving= 1 Carb chit, 1 Milk chit, 1 Protein chit, 1 Oil chit

CUCUMBER CHEESE-WITCH

2 palm size slices sprouted wheat bread	C
1/4 cup alfalfa sprouts	V
6 thin slices cucumber	V
1 slice natural swiss cheese (2 oz.)	M
1 t. mayonnaise	O

Spread mayonnaise on bread. Add cheese, cucumber and sprouts on one slice and cover with the other.
1 serving= 2 Carbohydrate chits, 1 Milk chit, 1 Oil chit

SALAD SUPREME

1 palm portion cheese, poultry or fish	**M or P**
red cabbage	**V**
green cabbage	**V**
carrots	**V**
celery	**V**
cucumbers	**V**
parsley	**V**
chard	**V**
collard greens	**V**
dandelion greens	**V**
kale	**V**
mustard greens	**V**
leeks	**V**
romaine lettuce	**V**
butter lettuce	**V**
red and green-leaf lettuce	**V**
mushrooms	**V**
onions or scallions	**V**
green pepper	**V**
radishes	**V**
spinach leaves	**V**
tomatoes	**V**
watercress	**V**
alfalfa sprouts	**V**
salad dressing	**O**

(I dare you to use them all!) From the above list select your favorite salad ingredients, tear, chop or cut and place in a large salad bowl. Avoid using iceberg lettuce. (It's too boring.) Add chopped broccoli or cauliflower for an interesting touch. Top your serving of greens with a palm-measured portion of sunflower seeds, chopped cheese, poultry or fish. Select a dressing.
1 serving= 1 Milk or Protein chit, 1 Oil, Unlimited Vegetable

MANHATTAN BUTTERMILK DRESSING

1 cup buttermilk	**M**
4 T. tomato or vegetable juice	**V**
1/4 t. dry mustard	**free**
1/4 t. garlic powder	**free**
1/4 t. lemon juice	**free**

Mix all ingredients in a glass container with tight cover. Chill. Shake before serving.
1/4 cup serving= 1 Milk chit

FINE FRENCH DRESSING

6 T. salad/vegetable oil	**O**
2 T. olive oil	**O**

1 T. rice vinegar	**free**
1 T. lemon juice	**free**
1/4 t. dry mustard	**free**
1 t. chopped scallions	**O**
1/4 t. basil	**V**
pinch of pepper	**free**
1 clove garlic	**V**

Place all ingredients in a glass container with tight fitting cover. Shake until thoroughly blended and chill. Allow garlic clove to sit in the bottle.
1 T. serving= 1 Oil chit

BLEU CHEESE DRESSING

2 oz. bleu cheese chunks	**M**
2 T. water	**free**
1 cup low-fat yogurt	**M**
2 T. parsley	**V**
1/4 t. onion powder	**V**

Stir by hand and chill in refrigerator. Keep in air tight container.
1/4 cup serving= 1 Milk chit

RUSSIAN DRESSING

1 can (8 1/4 oz.) stewed tomatoes plus liquid	**V**
1/2 cup cottage cheese (small curd)	**M**
3 T. pickle relish	**V**
2 T. rice vinegar	**free**

Mix together tomatoes and cottage cheese in a blender until smooth. Then, add pickle relish and vinegar and mix. Refrigerate and serve cold.
1/4 cup serving= 1 Milk chit

BREADS AND SPREADS

HEFTY WHEAT PANCAKES

1 cup whole wheat flour	**C**
1 t. double-acting baking powder	**free**
1 egg	**P**
1 T. honey	**O**
1 cup milk	**M**

Mix together all dry ingredients.   Mix egg and honey, then add milk. Combine dry and liquid mixtures. Use a lightly greased pan (or electric skillet set at   360 degrees) and turn over pancakes as soon as edges appear firm. Makes about 8 palm-sized pancakes. (Freeze leftovers and reheat by placing in toaster.)
1 pancake= 1 Carbohydrate chit

dr. Anne plan

RAISIN WHEAT WONDER

2 cups whole wheat/oat flour	C
1 t. baking soda	free
1 t. baking powder	free
1/2 t. salt	free
1/4 cup wheat germ	P
1/3 cup cooking oil	O
1 1/2 cups milk + 1 T. vinegar	M
1/2 cup honey or molasses	O
3/4 cup raisins	F
1 T. cinnamon	free
1 T. oats	C

Mix dry ingredients. Add honey to cooking oil, then mix with into soured milk. Mix liquid ingredients with dry ingredients. Let stand uncovered for about 20 minutes. Add raisins and cinnamon. Mix and pour batter into a greased loaf pan (about 9" X 5"). Sprinkle top with oats. Bake for 45 minutes at 400 degrees or until bread is browned and tests dry with a toothpick. Makes 1 loaf.

1 palm size, thumb thick serving= 1 Carbohydrate

PEASANT YEAST BREAD

1/4 cup cornmeal	C
3/4 cup warm water	free
2 packets (1/4 oz.) dry active yeast	free
1 T. baking powder	free
1 1/4 cups milk mixed with 1 1/2 T. lemon juice	M
5 cups whole wheat/oat flour	C

Mix warm water with yeast. Cover and let stand for 10 minutes. Add warmed soured milk and baking powder, and stir. Beat in 2 cups of flour for one minute. Cover bowl and let stand for 15 minutes. Slowly beat in remaining flour. Turn out dough on floured board and knead ten minutes or until smooth and elastic. Roll into round or desired shape and place on baking sheet that has been sprinkled with cornmeal. Bake for 30 minutes in preheated 350 degree oven. Makes 2 loaves.

1 palm size, thumb thick serving= 1 Carbohydrate chit

MOM HOYT'S SPECIAL SPREAD

1 cup cheddar cheese, shredded	M
1 can (6 oz.) crab meat	P
1 T. pickle relish	free
1/4 onion, diced	V
1/4 green pepper, diced	V
1 t. prepared mustard	free
2-3 rolls (cupped-palm size)	C

Preheat oven to 375 degrees. Mix crab, cheese, relish, onion, pepper and mustard. Slice rolls in half. Spread rounded 1- 11/2 T. of mixture on each half roll. Bake in oven for 15 minutes or until cheese starts to melt. (Can be served hot or cold.). Makes 2-3 servings.

1 roll serving= 1 Carbohydrate chit, 1 Protein chit

MAIN MEAL ENTREES

BAKED SALMON

2 palm size salmon filets/steaks	P
1/4 fresh cucumber, peeled	V
1 T. fresh parsley	V
1/4 lemon sliced without rind	free
1/2 t. dill weed	V

Place the salmon steak on a sheet of aluminum foil (large enough to wrap the fish). Place very thin cucumber and lemon slices, alternating, on top of fish. Garnish with parsley and dill. Wrap in the aluminum foil and bake for 25 minutes in a preheated 350 degree oven. (Or barbecue in the foil for 20 minutes.) Makes 2 servings.
1 serving= 1 Protein chit

CHICKEN BARBECUE BREAST

4 palm size chicken breasts or filets	P
1 clove garlic, minced	V
1/8 t. pepper	free
1/4 t. prepared mustard	free
1/2 t. lemon juice	free
1/4 t. dry mustard	free
1/2 cup tomato sauce or salsa	V

Remove skin from chicken and discard. Prepare the sauce, combining all ingredients and mix by hand. Baste the chicken with sauce and bake in a covered barbecue for 30 minutes. Baste again. Cook for another 15-20 minutes and serve. (Oven alternative: Bake in preheated 350 degree oven for 45 minutes.) Makes 4 servings.
1 serving=1 Protein chit

EGGPLANT PARMESAN

1 medium sized eggplant	V
1/4 cup mayonnaise	O
1/4 cup cornmeal	C
1 lb. mozzarella cheese	M
1 cup Italian cooking or herbed tomato sauce	V

Peel eggplant skin and cut in 1/2 inch slices. Spread mayonnaise thinly on each side of the eggplant slices and pat in cornmeal. Arrange slices on ungreased baking sheet. Bake at 425 degrees for 15 minutes. Then, top each slice with a tablespoon of cooking sauce and 1/2 thumb thick slice mozzarella cheese. Bake at 375 degrees for about 15 minutes or until cheese melts. Heat the remaining cooking sauce and pour over top after serving. Makes 4 servings.
1 serving= 1/2 Milk chit, 1 Oil chit, 1/2 Carbohydrate chit

dr. Anne plan

BRUSSELS SPROUTS SOUFFLE

1/4 cup butter or margarine	O
1/4 cup whole wheat or oat flour	C
1 cup milk	M
4 egg yolks	P
4 egg whites	P
4 oz. cheddar cheese shredded	M
2 cups cooked Brussels sprouts, chopped	V

Melt butter and blend in the flour. Add milk and cook until mixture thickens, stirring constantly for white sauce. Remove from heat. Beat egg yolks until thick and lemon-colored. Slowly blend the egg yolks into the white sauce and stir rapidly. Add in shredded cheese, finely chopped Brussels sprouts. Beat egg whites until stiff, but not dry; fold into mixture. Pour into an ungreased 2-quart souffle dish. Bake in moderate oven, 350 degrees, for 40 minutes or until knife inserted comes our clean. Makes 4 servings.
1 serving or 2 cupped palms= 1 Protein chit, 1 Milk chit

WHITE SAUCE

1 t. butter or margarine	O	
1 T. enriched white flour	C	
1/2 cup milk (at least 2% fat)	M	(optional: 1 T. mixed
carrots and peas)	V/C	

Melt butter in saucepan. Remove from heat and mix in flour. Slowly add milk over heat and bring to slow boil for about one minute, mixing constantly until thickened. (Add carrots and peas.) Serve immediately. Makes 1 serving.
1 serving= 1 Milk chit, 1 Oil chit

MOTHER'S VEGETABLE COMBINATION DISH

4 cups vegetables in season (broccoli, squash, carrots, etc.)	V
1/2 cup natural cheddar cheese, shredded	M
1/2 cup brown rice	C

Cook brown rice and let stand. Steam vegetables for about 15 minutes until just tender. Place the hot vegetables in the center of a large serving place and top with the shredded cheese. While cheese is melting ring the vegetables with rice. Serve immediately. Makes 2 servings.
1 serving= 1 Carbohydrate chit, 1 Milk chit

SHEPHERD'S POT LUCK

1/2 cup leftover meat	P
2 cups assorted vegetables plus onion	V
1 can V-8 juice/ tomato juice	V
1/4 cup milk	M
pepper, garlic to taste	free
1 t. Worcestershire sauce	free
2 palm-size potatoes mashed	C
paprika	free

Preheat oven to 375 degrees. In 11/2 quart casserole dish combine meat, vegetables, onion, pepper and Worcestershire sauce. Pat down evenly in dish. Make mashed potatoes by cooking, mashing and mixing with 2 t. butter and 1/4 cup milk. Place tablespoons of mashed potatoes on top and spread to cover mixture. Sprinkle with paprika. Bake 40 minutes or until golden brown and bubbly. Makes 2 servings.
1 serving= 1 Protein chit, 1 Carbohydrate chit, 1 Oil chit

MEATLESS MOUSSAKA

1/2 onion, chopped	V
1 T. parsley	V
1/4 t. pepper	free
1/4 t. nutmeg	free
1 can (16 oz.) tomatoes, drained	V
1/4 cup seasoned tomato sauce	V
1 large eggplant, long shape	V
4 eggs	P
1/2 cup milk	M
1 cup mozzarella cheese, grated	M
1 t. cooking oil	O

Peel and thinly slice eggplant. Put half of slices on bottom of lightly greased 2-quart casserole. Brown the onion in oil and add to mixture of tomatoes, tomato sauce, milk, parsley, pepper and nutmeg. Pour mixture over eggplant slices. Place remaining eggplant slices on top. Cover and bake for 30 minutes in a 375 degree oven. Beat the eggs and stir into warm, not hot casserole. Top with cheese and bake uncovered for 15 minutes or more. Makes 4 servings.
1 serving= 1 Protein chit, 1 Milk chit

CHILI A LA LOUISE

2 cups red kidney beans	P
1 onion, chopped	V
1 garlic clove, chopped	V
1 sprig parsley	V
1 bay leaf	free
1/4 t. salt	free
1 t. cooking oil	O
1/4 green pepper, chopped	V
3/4 cup bean liquid	free
1 t. chili powder	free
1/4 t. red cayenne pepper	
4 tomatoes, chopped	V
1 cup celery chopped	V

Rinse beans and let stand overnight in a pot filled with 4 cups of water. Add 1/4 onion, garlic, parsley, bay leaf and salt to the soaking water, cover and simmer 1 hour until the beans are tender. Drain the solids from the liquid, retaining 3/4 cup bean liquid. Remove bay leaf and parsley sprig. Saute 1/2 onion and green pepper in cooking oil until slightly browned. Remove from heat. Add back bean liquid; then add chili powder, red pepper, chopped tomatoes and celery. Stir in kidney beans. Simmer mixture over low heat for at least 45 minutes. Makes 4 servings.
1 serving= 1 Protein chit

BAKED POTATO PROUD

1 cupped palm Russet potato	C
2 T. sour cream or yogurt	M
1 T. chives	V
dash pepper	free

Bake potato in 425 degree oven for about 45 minutes. Cut an "X" across the top and puff up the potato by pushing the sides towards the center. Create an indention in the middle and fill with sour cream or yogurt and chives, then add pepper. Makes 1 serving.
1 serving= 1 Carbohydrate chit, 1 Milk chit

TURKEY BREAST BAKE

4 oz. turkey breast slices	P
1/4 cup corn meal	C
2 t. prepared mustard	free
2 oz. mozzarella cheese	M
dash pepper	free

Lightly spread mustard on turkey slices and pat in corn meal. Place on cooking sheet and bake in preheated 450 degree oven for 10 minutes. Top with mozzarella cheese and a dash of pepper. Return to oven for another 5 minutes or until cheese is melted. Makes 1 serving.
1 serving= 1 Protein chit, 1 Milk chit

DESSERTS

BLUEBERRY COBBLER

1 cup whole wheat/oat flour	C
1 1/2 t. baking powder	free
1/4 t. salt	free
12 oz. blueberries	F
1 t. lemon juice	free
1/2 cup water	free
1/4 cup butter or margarine, soft	O
1 egg slightly beaten	P
1/2 cup milk	M
1 1/2 t. vanilla	free

Mix flour, baking powder and salt. Mix egg, milk and vanilla, then add butter. Combine dry and liquid ingredients slowly mixing and beating them well. Pour blueberries, water and lemon juice mixture in bottom of 11/2 greased quart casserole. Spoon batter over top. Bake for 30 minutes in preheated 375 degree oven. Makes 4 servings.
1 serving or two 1/3 cup palms= 1 Fruit chit, 1 Carb chit

dr. Anne plan

DEBBIE'S DELIGHT COOKIES

1 1/2 cups whole wheat/oat flour	**C**
1/2 cup bran	**C**
1 3/4 cups old fashioned oats	**C**
1/2 t. baking soda	**free**
1/2 t. salt	**free**
1/4 cup cooking oil	**free**
1/2 cup honey/brown sugar	**O**
1 egg ,well beaten	**P**
1 t. vanilla	**free**
1/2 cup chopped walnuts	**P**
1 cup mashed over-ripe banana	
(or applesauce, cooked squash/ pumpkin)	**F or V**
1/2 cup raisins	**F**

Mix all dry ingredients. Then add all mixed liquids and include banana, walnuts and raisins. Place batter in rounded tablespoons on greased cookie sheet. Bake for 15 minutes in 350 degree oven. Makes about 5 dozen cookies (textured and crunchy).
2 cookies= 1 Carbohydrate chit

COCO MOUSSE

1 envelope (1T.) unflavored gelatin	**P**
1 can (13 oz.)evaporated skimmed milk	**M**
2 T. cocoa (unsweetened)	**free**
1 T. dark brown sugar	**O**
1 t. vanilla extract	**free**
(optional: 1/4 t. mint extract)	**free**

Mix cocoa and sugar in 1/4 cup milk until blended. In a medium saucepan gradually sprinkle gelatin over remainder of milk, cooking over low heat and stirring until gelatin is dissolved. Add cocoa mixture and stir until blended. Pour the mixture into a 11/2 quart mixing bowl and set aside to cool (or place in refrigerator about 15 minutes). Add vanilla. (Add mint.) Beat at high speed with electric mixer until thick and foamy. Place in covered container and refrigerate until firm. (Or store in freezer. Allow 20 minutes to defrost.) Makes 4 servings.
1 serving= 1 Milk chit

FRUIT AND CHEESE BOARD

sliced fresh pineapple	**F**
green/red/black seedless grapes	**F**
sliced red delicious apples	**F**
low-fat cheddar cheese	**M**
farmer's cheese	**M**

Arrange on a platter wood board, slice apple and pineapple. Accent with small bunches of grapes. Put cheese slices to one side and eat in combination with fruit.
1 cupped-palm serving= 1 Fruit chit
1 palm size, thumb thick cheese or 2 oz.= 1 Milk chit

Appendix C

Practice Circles for Support

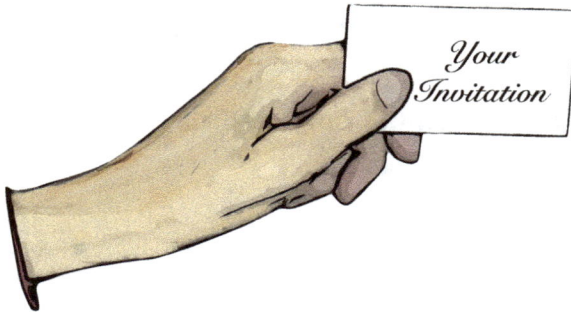

About the dr.Anne Association

Knowing what to do, what foods to eat and how to monitor portions is essential. However, a helping hand to maintain good lifestyle habits is often crucial for success. To this end the dr.Anne Association assists Practice Circles to bring people together who are interested in mutual support. People like yourself can find or form a Practice Circle.

A Practice Circles operate across the country using a format similar to the one described below. Use this format to form your own self-help Practice Circle. Our goal is to make this fun and easy! The basics are given below:

How to Form a Practice Circle

Here are the steps to follow:

First, you will need to form a **T E A M**:

Three At Least	Active members to form a group
Experience	Knowledge using the MagicHand
Administrative	Keeping in touch with members
Meeting space	A regular place/time to meet

Then find a way to meet. This could be either in-person (a home, meeting room, or cafe) or online (via Zoom, Zoho or other internet venue). Establish a time when at least 3 people can meet for about 45 minutes regularly. Eventually through social media or notices others will join you. We recommend one Point for review and discussion a week.

Next, select officers Here are **The Three Linking Hands** for designating responsibilities

Ruling-Hand: Contact number and/or email for the Circle.

Right-Hand: Assists Ruling-Hand, organizes events.

Post-Hand: Meeting notices. Donations for expenses.

If desired: Create a space for your Practice Circle on social media. *Why is it called a Practice Circle?* <u>New members can enter at any time</u>. Points continue, one meeting to the next, and repeat again. Like a circle, practice and learning are never ending!

129

dr. Anne plan

How to conduct the Meeting:

Sections <u>Apportion</u>, <u>Move</u>, and <u>Silence</u> each include three chapters called Points: a total of nine chapter Points. Focus on one Point each meeting using the Practice Point questions in this book to stimulate discussion. The following meeting then focuses on the next Practice Point and so on sequentially. After reaching Point 9, start over again at Point 1! Keep it going.

The MagicSquare card shows Practice Points Completed:

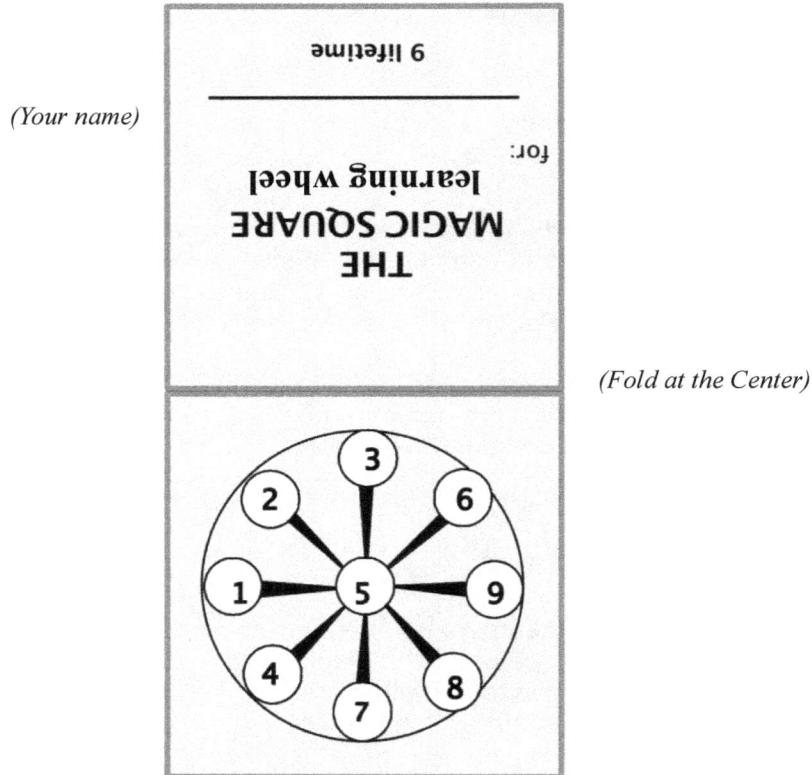

(Your name)

(Fold at the Center)

What is the MagicSquare? Did you notice that on each Practice page there was a circle in the upper right corner displaying the Point number? That was not just for decoration!

Looking at the MagicSquare card, all nine Point numbers are shown in the learning wheel. Each line when added across sums 15. That just happens to be the "magic number" of chits allotted each day! (And we did that just for fun with mathematics).

You can copy this MagicSquare card to use at in-person Practice Circle meetings. Use heavy paper, fold, and place the fold-over card in front of you so others can see your name. Then as you complete each Practice Point, use a pen to fill in the Point dot on your MagicSquare card.

dr. Anne plan

When all 9 Point PRACTICES are completed and the 9 dots are now filled, you have accomplished the program. Congratulations! As you continue to repeat the course, even more will be learned.

What happens in the Practice Circle
Sample videos showing what takes place in the Practice Circle are on Dr. Anne's YouTube channel. Video your sessions and they might be posted on that channel to share with others.

For more information
The www.dranne.org website provides a Practice Circle section with links. Program updates and more detailed session guidelines are available there as well.

Start at any Point and complete all Nine Points. Then continue to repeat Points!

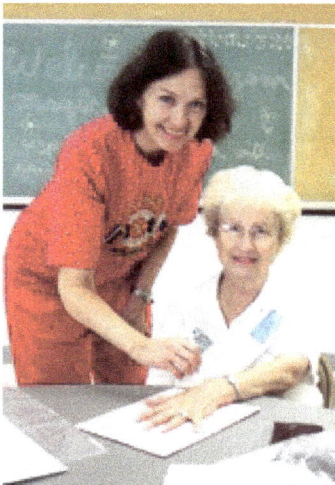

Drawing the MagicHand

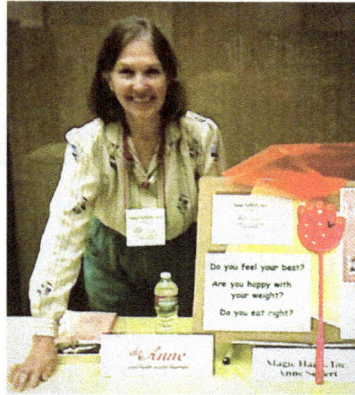

dr.Anne speaking at Hollywood Screen Actor's Guild Health Fair

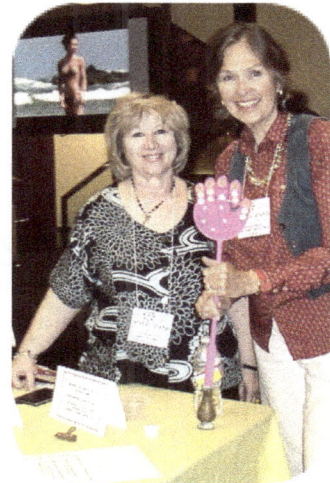

Inviting new members with Sandra

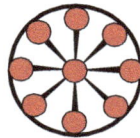

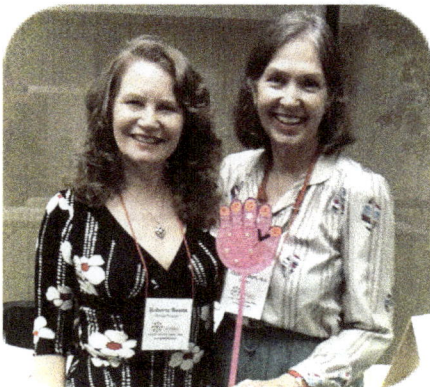

Actress Roberta Bassin lends a hand

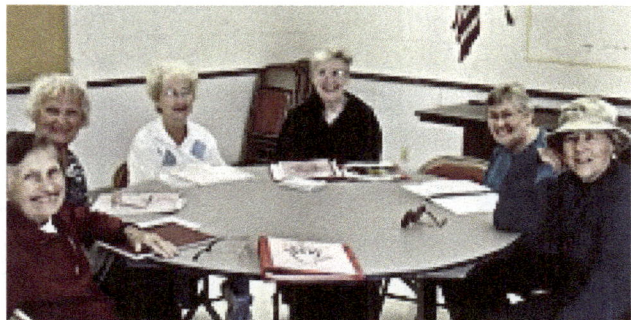

Practice Circle in action with Guide Marilyn

<h1>Appendix D</h1>

MagicHand Chits Page

Here's another way to Count Chits!

Copy this weekly Chit tally & carry it with you— or add to your smartphone.

DAY	Milk			Fruit			Carbs			Protein			Oils			Veggies		
Chits	1	2	3	1	2	3	1	2	3	1	2	3	1	2	3	Unlimited		
Mon.																		
Tues.																		
Wed.																		
Thu.																		
Fri.																		
Sat.																		
Sun.																		

Start with 21-Days & keep going for Life!

Check the box for each chit used. Place a "O" next to the DAY if you go over 15 chits.. Place a strike (/) through the DAY when at or within the allotted 15 chits-- 12 palms and 3 thumbs. Vegetables are unlimited.

DAY	Milk 1. 2. 3			Fruit 1. 2. 3			Carbs 1. 2. 3			Protein 1. 2. 3			Oils 1. 2. 3			Veggies 1. 2. 3		
1																		
2																		
3																		
4																		
5																		
6																		
7																		
8																		
9																		
10																		
11																		
12																		
13																		
14																		
15																		
16																		
17																		
18																		
19																		
20																		
21																		

Appendix E
Seeing Fingers on your MagicHand

These lists give you a good idea of what foods fall into various food group categories. Some foods can be counted under more than one food group. Note that even though botanically a tomato is a fruit, we count it as a Vegetable. You will also find other nuances within groups.

MILK & DAIRY PRODUCTS *(palm/cupped portion)*	*If allergic to Milk & Dairy, below are substitutes high in calcium (use Milk chits for these instead)*
Buttermilk	*Almonds*
Camembert	*Canned mackerel*
Cheddar, Farmer's cheese	*Canned salmon*
Cottage cheese	*Canned sardines*
Cream cheese/Neufchatel	*Chickpeas (garbanzo beans)*
Hoop cheese/ Feta cheese	*Dried figs*
Ice cream/Ice milk	*Filberts*
Milk: whole, 2%, skim	*Fortified bread*
Parmesan	*Oats, Oatmeal*
Pudding/custard	*Pistachio nuts*
Swiss cheese	*Red or white pinto beans*
Whipped cream	*Sesame seed*
Yogurt, Kefir	Tofu

High Calcium: Unlimited Foods

Beets	Okra
Broccoli	Parsley
Mustard, collard, turnip greens	Spinach, Kale

FRUIT & FRUIT JUICES	*(palm/cupped portion)*
Apples	Oranges
Apricots	Peaches
Avocado	Pears
Bananas	Persimmons
Berries	Pineapple
Cantaloupe	Plantain
Cherries	Plums
Cranberries	Pomegranate
Dates	Prunes
Figs	Raisins
Fruit pies	Raspberries
Grapefruit	Strawberries
Grapes	Tangerine
Kiwi fruit	Watermelon
Lemons and limes	Wine
Mandarins	
Mangos	
Melons	
Nectarines	
Olives	

CARBOHYDRATES & STARCHY VEGETABLES *(palm/cupped portion)*

Bagels	Lentils
Barley	Millet
Beans: black, kidney, lima, navy, pinto	Muffins
Beer	Oatmeal
Biscuits	Pancakes, waffles
Bran	Parsnip
Breads, rolls	Pasta
Buckwheat	Peas
Cakes, jello	Pita
Cereals	Plantain
Chickpeas	Popcorn
Cookies	Potatoes (all), potato chips
Corn, popcorn	Pretzels
Crackers, croutons	Pumpkin, Yams
Croissants	Rice, rice cakes
Danish pastry	Rye
Doughnuts, cupcakes	Stuffing, bread/rice based
Edamame	Taro
English muffins, crumpets	Tortillas,, tortilla chips
Grits	Wheat
Ice cream cone	Winter squash: acorn, butternut

PROTEIN SOURCES *(palm portion)*

Almonds	Navy beans
Beef	Nuts, most varieties
Black beans	Organ meats
Cheese/ Feta cheese	Peanuts
Chia, poppy seeds	Pecans
Chicken	Pinto beans
Cold cuts	Pistachios
Duck	Pork
Edamame	Pumpkin seeds
Eggs	Sausages/ frankfurters
Filberts	Shellfish: clams, crab, lobster, shrimp, etc.
Fish: flounder, herring, salmon, sardines, tuna, etc.	Soybeans, tempeh
Game	Sunflower seeds
Goose	Tofu
Green peas	Turkey
Kidney beans	Veal
Lamb	Walnuts
Lentils	Wheat germ
Lima beans	Yogurt
Liver	
Lox/Smoked fish	
Macadamia nuts	

OILS & FATS AND CONCENTRATED SUGARS *(thumb measure)*

Barbeque sauce	
Butter/Margarine	
Caramel	
Chocolate fudge	
Chocolates	
Coconut oil	
Gravy (oil-base)	
Hard candy	
Ice cream syrup	
Jams and jellies, preserves	
Mayonnaise	
Molasses, Honey	
Nut and seed butters	
Pancake syrup/ maple syrup	
Peanut butter	
Salad dressing	
Sweet sauces, toppings, etc.	
Vegetable oils	

VEGETABLES & HERBS *(unlimited)*

Artichokes	Green, red chilies
Arugula	Green, yellow string beans
Asparagus	Herbs, all
Bamboo shoots	Horseradish
Bay leaf	Jicama
Bean sprouts	Kale
Beets	Kimchi
Bok choy	Leeks
Broccoli	Mushrooms (all)
Brussels Sprouts	Mustard greens
Cabbage (all)	Okra
Carrots, alfalfa sprouts	Olives
Cauliflower	Onions
Celery	Parsley
Chard	Peppers
Chayote	Pickles
Cilantro	Radishes
Cucumbers	Rhubarb
Eggplant	Rutabaga
Endive	Salad greens, lettuce (all)
Escarole	Salsa/Picante
Fennel	Sauerkraut
Garlic	

VEGETABLES & HERBS *(continued)*

Scallions	Tomatoes
Seaweed (all)	Turnips
Shallots	Vegetable juices
Snap peas, snow peas	Water chestnuts
Spices	Watercress
Spinach	Zucchini
Sprouts	
Squash: summer, spaghetti	
Sun chokes	

& Free to use:

baking powder, baking soda	lemon juice, vinegar
chili powder, Worstershire	salt, pepper,
cocoa (unsweetened)	soy sauce, teriyaki
coffee, tea	water, mineral water
flavorings, vanilla	yeast
ketchup, mustard	

Anything missing?
Feel free to add to these lists.

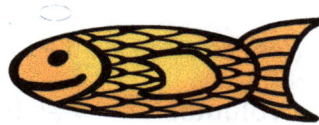

Give a man a fish and
you feed him for a day

Teach a man to fish and
you feed him for a lifetime

---Lao Tzu
Chinese Proverb

A letter to you from dr.Anne

Dear Reader,

You have completed the learning part of this Plan. I applaud you for taking this step. You probably already realize that you can't just stop here! Practice Points need reinforcement in order for you to reach and maintain your goals. How are you going to help yourself? Is there a way to keep motivated while helping others at the same time?

Wouldn't you like to keep going, and to keep practicing, with others, to share and enjoy their support? Here's how our dr.Anne Association is structured so that you can do just that.

You can lead your own group! Yes, become a **V I P!**

Practice Circles can be led by a **Volunteer**, or by an **Independent** coach or in **Partnership** with other organizations, clubs, and sponsors. This is something you can do in your spare time to maybe earn money for yourself or benefit a club and others.

As a VOLUNTEER: *if you want a self-help support option*

You can start your own Practice Circle in your neighborhood, or online. You become the Guide, organize the Circle, and create sessions free of charge with other volunteers to assist.

As an INDEPENDENT coach: *if you are a health professional*

You can become a Guide and offer Practice Circles as part of your practice. Some licensing by the Association may be required.

As a PARTNER: *if you have an existing non-profit organization or club or business*

You can offer this program to your members or employees. Also, we can work together on mutually beneficial fund raising projects.

You may be wondering how it is that we can control what happens in our Practice Circles. For every V I P we have a written protocol for our Practice Circle sessions. Mostly we work on the honor system since there is no reason to change the order or content of our program. It has been tested for decades and it works.

If you are interested in becoming part of the **TEAM** as a **VIP** then please let us know. We are here to help you and to help others find good health, happiness and weight control!

Once you have organized your Circle, we ask that you register with the *dr.Anne Association* so that you will receive free updates and advice. If desired we will include you in our Registry of Practice Circles so that others may join your group.

With your leadership the Association can accomplish its mission to provide an easy to learn and easy to use program for good health.

We encourage those interested in keeping their weight under control to get involved-- to **GET, GUIDE, & GROW** by following these three steps to become part of the VIP TEAM.

1. **GET** the materials needed to instruct the dr.Anne plan

2. **GUIDE** a Practice Circle as a Volunteer, Independent coach or Partner

3. **GROW** your Practice Circle through social media and outreach.

You may be wondering what the qualifications are to lead a Practice Circle. In general, after you have completed all nine Points of the program either as a home study project or in a Practice Circle, you can elect to stay active in the program. You can form your own Circle Group and become a Guide. With Practice you will become better and better as a Guide. And we are here to assist if needed.

If you do not want to create your own Practice Circle we can help you find an online Circle to join. Make sure you have the program book or other format materials. You may enter an on-going Practice Circle at any time since the Points repeat. dr.Anne Plan materials are available online, but Independent and Partner program fees may vary due to sponsoring organization and professional instruction charges. No auditing is permitted or guests allowed unless authorized by the Guide.

Please let us know if you want to become a part of our Association. Our Memberships last for a lifetime! To reach me please visit our website at www.dranne.org and you will be directed from there. Thanks.

All good wishes and I hope to hear from you!
dr.Anne

July 4, 2025

dr. Anne plan

144

www.ingramcontent.com/pod-product-compliance
Lightning Source LLC
Chambersburg PA
CBHW080616270326
41928CB00016B/3085